AUTOMATION OF CLINICAL
ELECTROENCEPHALOGRAPHY

A CONFERENCE

PARTICIPANTS

R. G. Bickford
N. Burch
J. R. G. Carrie
G. Dumermuth
J. D. Frost, Jr.
I. Hagne
E. Kaiser
P. Kellaway
L. E. Larsen
A. H. Levy
R. Magnusson
R. L. Maulsby
K. E. Morander
J. Persson
I. Petersén
A. Remond
R. L. Roessler
B. Saltzberg
D. O. Walter
S. S. Viglione
L. H. Zetterberg

This conference was sponsored by The Methodist Hospital, Houston, Texas. The Editors are grateful to Mr. Ted Bowen, President, and to the Board of Trustees of the Methodist Hospital for their generous support.

Automation of Clinical Electroencephalography

Editors:

Peter Kellaway
Professor of Physiology, Baylor College of Medicine,
Chief of Service, Neurophysiology,
The Methodist Hospital
Houston, Texas, U.S.A.

Ingemar Petersén
Department of Clinical Neurophysiology
The Sahlgren Hospital
Göteborg, Sweden

Raven Press, Publishers ▪ New York

Made in the United States of America.

International Standard Book Number
0–911216–45–6
Library of Congress Catalog Card Number
72–96334

Preface

The large quantity of data which EEG recordings produce is of fundamental importance to clinical electroencephalography but at the same time poses a problem for the clinical electroencephalographer who must interpret individual EEG records and provide diagnostic guidance for the referring physicians. Even greater problems are presented by the increased amount of data that is amassed when several EEG traces from the same patient must be compared and when EEG recordings from entire patient groups must be compared with those from other patient groups or from control groups. Thus it is not surprising that the need has long been felt for methods of automatic analysis that would provide an objective description of EEG records by electronic means. Several such methods, dealing with correlation analysis, spectral analysis and pattern recognition, have been in use for varying periods of time, but the hopes raised by these methods centered initially on the possibility of enhancing the study of physiological or pathophysiological processes and mechanisms. A great deal of work has been published in these fields, and although there has been general disappointment over the reported results, no penetrating critical analysis has yet been made of the subject.

Although automatic EEG analysis has long been a subject of interest, the possibility of automatic EEG interpretation has been almost completely ignored. Automatic interpretation of the clinical EEG offers an attractive prospect from many points of view, not the least of which is that it would provide an objective evaluation of the EEG. Further, automatic EEG interpretation would free the well-trained neurophysiologist from the drudgery of evaluating a large number of easily classifiable EEGs and would enable him to spend his time on problems that make full use of his expertise.

These ideas were raised in the early 1960's by the Department of Clinical Neurophysiology in Göteborg, which, with the Kaiser Laboratories in Copenhagen, was then developing methods for automatic EEG analyses, especially spectral analysis, correlation analysis in the form of reverse correlation and, subsequently, for EEG pattern recognition. This group proposed the idea of establishing EEG centers, *i.e.,* technically well-equipped central EEG laboratories in which qualified physicians and technicians could supervise and monitor computer-based interpretation of EEG signals transmitted by mail, telephone, or some other system for EEG signal telemetry from satellite laboratories located some distance from the central laboratory. The telemetry of EEG recordings from peripheral to central units opens up the possibility of developing service activities at the central units in order to provide rapid diagnostic results to meet the needs of peripheral units. These views predominate in a long-range medical and technical project that is currently being undertaken as a collaborative effort of the Department of Clinical Neurophysiology in Göteberg, the Kaiser Laboratory in Copenhagen, and the Department of Applied Electronics, Chalmers Institute of Technology, Göteborg.

The present conference on the automation of clinical electroencephalography grew out of discussions between Drs. Kellaway and Petersén, whose departments at Göteborg and in Houston, Texas, have collaborated since the late 1950's and who have long been interested in the development of methods of automatic analysis of clinical electroencephalography.

The purpose of this conference, which was the first of its kind, was to bring together a group of internationally distinguished technical experts in spectral analysis, wavelength analysis, and pattern recognition, and several experts in clinical neurophysiology so that they could discuss the possibility of transmitting EEG signals, report on their methods for the analysis of EEG signals, and discuss the possibility of applying these methods with a view toward the creation of the EEG centers described above. Although the discussions reflected the tentative, preliminary character of research in the field, the participants were unanimously in favor of pursuing the aims of the conference, the development of methods for automatic interpretation of EEGs and the continuation of discussions on the possibility of establishing a system of centers for the automatic evaluation of EEGs.

Ingemar Petersén
Göteborg, 1971

Contents

Automation of Clinical Electroencephalography.
Edited by P. Kellaway and I. Petersén.
Raven Press, New York © 1973.

Automation of Clinical Electroencephalography: The Nature and Scope of the Problem

Peter Kellaway

Department of Neurophysiology, The Methodist Hospital, and Baylor College of Medicine, Houston, Texas 77025

This volume is directed specifically to the problem of automation of clinical electroencephalography. Some of the participants, notably Drs. Petersén and Kaiser and their colleagues in Sweden and Denmark and Dr. Bickford in the United States, have been deeply involved in the development of research along these lines. In 1967, Drs. Walter and Brazier conducted a workshop, *Advances in EEG Analysis,* which was the first conference to consider the implications for the clinical electroencephalographer of the then recent efforts in statistical and computerized study of the EEG. Previously, mathematicians and computer scientists had been reluctant to consider the problems of applied research in electroencephalography, and most efforts in the field of automation of EEG analysis had been devoted with more or less success to research into the fundamental brain processes rather than to the urgent needs of clinical electroencephalography.

It is the purpose of this chapter to demonstrate the scope and complexity of the problems confronting the scientist interested in the automation of clinical electroencephalography and to emphasize the need for imaginative applied research as well as the ultimate value of its results.

At this time, most of the necessary techniques have already been developed, and it remains for these techniques to be applied appropriately in order to accomplish the task at hand. Appropriately is, of course, the key word. It is a common dictum of computer scientists that any problem that

1

can be adequately specified can be resolved with the use of the appropriate computer. The fundamental difficulties in EEG have been that the specification of the task has often been inadequate and that the automatic techniques of analysis and characterization have been focused on unitary or limited aspects of the data. The appropriate approach to the automation of clinical electroencephalography might be to ascertain first how the human "computer" deals with the visual data and then, if not to simulate the process, at least to recognize and to evaluate each aspect of the process for its heuristic significance.

Simulation is a reputable technique in computer and mathematical science. The empirical approach of visual analysis has been remarkably productive when we consider that it can yield, for example, an accurate assessment of conceptual age, the cause of a state of altered consciousness, and the approximate site of a discrete lesion, or it can signal the occurrence of brain insult during surgery. If computer analysis were only to simulate the process of visual analysis, adding those important features of the nonbiological computer, consistency and quantification, much would be accomplished. Furthermore, our experience with the development of automatic sleep staging indicates that a continuing interaction between visual and computer analysis enables the electroencephalographer to recognize which information ought to be analyzed as well as to understand how his own biological computer operates. Electroencephalography has proved a useful and often indispensable tool of clinical diagnosis, but its development has gone as far as is possible without quantitation and more precise characterization of the data. We must give numbers to what are now largely expressed as impressions if the potentialities of EEG in clinical medicine are to be realized fully.

Automation and telemetry techniques can provide reliable clinical electroencephalography to greater numbers of people at decreased cost. Adequate and reliable diagnostic services are readily available only to a small segment of the world's population, not only in medically underdeveloped continents such as Africa, Asia, and South America but also in the United States, where approximately 7,000 clinical EEG laboratories operate but fail to meet the needs of the population, particularly in lower income and rural areas. In addition, there are probably fewer than 200 adequately trained electroencephalographers to serve the entire U.S. population of 210 million. Consequently, most clinical electroencephalography in the United States is substandard, and it is not generally known to most referring physicians that they are not receiving the diagnostic aid that they should expect from EEG studies. At the same time, substandard laboratories continue to multiply because of an ever-increasing demand for diagnostic EEG services.

That poor electroencephalography may confound or even controvert good clinical evaluation is often obscured by a blind acceptance of the "objective" information obtained by the machine. The all-important consideration — the skill and experience required to interpret the EEG information or even to ensure good data — is neglected because of the pressure to fill the need. This pressure is compounded of financial considerations and the need that most hospitals feel to have all the modern facilities. The absurdity of providing modern diagnostic facilities in the absence of adequately trained personnel may be illustrated by a case in point, that of a laboratory in a small city in Texas which is representative of many throughout the country. Here nearly every child referred is found to have an abnormal EEG, and the usual clinical interpretation is that the abnormality is consistent with a convulsive disorder. This type of situation, common in this country, obviously serves no constructive purpose and is in fact harmful medically, sociologically, and in terms of possible medical-legal consequences for the patients and their relatives. In many such laboratories, the technical quality of the recordings is such as to preclude reliable interpretation, and the clinical diagnostic impressions, which are rendered often without benefit of reliable clinical information, may be inappropriate and misleading.

The needs to improve the precision and scope of diagnostic electroencephalography and to increase the availability of reliable clinical EEGs are interrelated. As computer techniques of quantification and precise characterization of EEG activity tend to standardize criteria of normality and abnormality, improve reliability, and expand the diagnostic utility of electroencephalography, so too will the demand burgeon and the pressure to meet this demand increase.

The financial requirements of establishing a large number of individual, fully equipped, computerized laboratories stagger the imagination, and the problems of providing this multitude with qualified electroencephalographers seem to be beyond resolution. It appears to us that central computerized EEG facilities to serve communities are a reasonable and practical solution. Such central facilities would, in addition to their own in-house EEG activities, service satellite laboratories in adjacent and outlying districts. The extent of the latter would be dependent upon such considerations as the size of the population to be served.

Many major medical centers provide an environment to test in microcosm a model of a central laboratory with satellite facilities. Such models permit evaluation of the economic as well as the technical aspects of such operations before commitments to any particular system or systems, for example, of telemetry, are made. The newborn nursery, the emergency room, the surgical operating room suites, and the intensive care facilities provide the basis of a model of varying complexity for a satellite system operated from a central EEG laboratory. Each of these various types of satellite unit affords different types of problems with regard to such questions as the degree of participation of the technologist in the data acquisition and analysis loop, the extent of pre-processing to be carried out at the site, and the relative merits of special hardware versus general computer use for various types of tasks.

All of these considerations constitute the background for this volume. Its organization and frame of reference developed from the organizers' long-term concern for more precise criteria for EEG diagnosis, especially in children, and our recognition of the limitations of impressionistic and idiosyncratic evaluation of EEG data. The potentialities of clinical and research electroencephalography cannot be realized until such impressions are replaced with numbers and subjective descriptions replaced with mathematically derived characterizations. Finally, the ever-increasing demand for clinical electroencephalography is not currently being fulfilled and will only be met through the most advanced technological developments.

The practical problem of finding adequate financial support for such applied research and for its implementation should be resolved without difficulty since health-care delivery is today a major concern of responsible local, national, and international governments. Changing patterns of medical practice and of the methods of payment for services rendered and the ever-present need to provide adequate medical care to all segments of the population make it mandatory to move mightily in this direction for all types of laboratory diagnostic services. Electroencephalography represents only one very small part of the total problem of adequate health-care delivery, but it is our part, and solution of the problem in this quite complex area might well serve as a general model for effective delivery of laboratory services.

PROGRAMMING THE BIOLOGICAL COMPUTER: A GUIDE FOR AUTOMATIC ANALYSIS?

Progress in the automation of clinical electroencephalography has been hampered most by the inability of the electroencephalographer to communicate the steps in his visual analysis of an EEG. Clinical electroencephalographers do not always know precisely how they arrive at their diagnostic impressions, and, indeed, the "pattern-reading" school of clinical electroencephalography has clothed the subjective process with a certain mystique in which the derivation of the diagnostic impression appears as a gestalt—a revelation without benefit of organized and clearly defined steps of analysis.

However, the "reading" of an EEG can in fact be an orderly and rational process with a logical progression to a final evaluation, as illustrated very briefly in the Appendix. The steps in the visual analysis can be specified and therefore can be replicated by computer methods. On the other hand, expressions such as a "spikey pattern" or "pattern of immature character" are so imprecise as to defy computer analysis and are therefore useless.

There are many ways in which the human EEG can be characterized analytically. The analysis system which I am about to describe has been the basis of my own practice and has proved useful as a didactic tool during the past 25 years. The outline of the steps of visual analysis which follows was prepared for the engineers and computer scientists — it is not meant for expert electroencephalographers for whom there will be nothing new.

Age and State

The visual analysis of the EEG begins with two crucial, "extrinsic" entries: the age of the patient and his state of alertness and of general well-being. It would seem obvious that these two factors should be considered, but many EEG analyses have not been controlled for state, especially in children, where not only the alertness but the affective state of the child may influence the EEG pattern, as Maulsby (1971) and others before him have shown (Faure, 1950a, b; Walter, 1950; Melin, 1953; Garsche, 1956; Lairy, 1956).

An effective system of automation requires that the data be acquired under programmed control; in other words, it is necessary to control the situation and stimulus field in a manner appropriate to the age and clinical status of the patient and to provide the technician with instructions programmed on the basis of the ongoing data or possibly on the basis of some preprocessing of the data at the site.

Elements of Visual Analysis

Once the age and state of the patient are entered, any electrical activity of cerebral origin is characterized in terms of each of the following parameters: (1) frequency or wavelength; (2) voltage; (3) locus; (4) wave form; (5) interhemispheric coherence (i.e., voltage and frequency and symmetry/synchrony on the two sides) (6) character of wave occurrence (random, serial, continuous) (7) regulation (voltage and frequency) (8) reactivity.

In visual analysis, all of these factors and their interrelationships are taken into account in order to arrive at an evaluation. Automatic analysis must consider all of these factors and their interrelationship or establish those which are essential to achieving an evaluation of equal or better significance. A system of analysis which deals with a single parameter, such as frequency, or even a combination of two parameters, such as in power-spectral analysis, can have only limited usefulness, and indeed this proved to be the case. For instance, the significance of a certain power spectrum will be determined by the age and the state of the subject, by its location or field on the head, and, very importantly, by the manner of occurrence of the individual wave components. The normal adult electrogram awake is characterized by a predominant rhythmic activity in the occipital region which is variously designated the Berger rhythm, the occipital alpha rhythm, or sometimes, loosely, the "alpha rhythm."

The presence and characteristics of this rhythm are central to the evaluation of the EEG. For example, the degree of abnormality of a record with much random, high voltage, 3 to 5 per second activity in anterior head regions is very much affected by the presence or absence of a normal occipital alpha rhythm. The absence of an occipital rhythm of normal alpha frequency renders the electrogram much more abnormal and its significance more ominous. Similarly, the presence of a sustained 5 per second rhythm in the central region bilaterally is not considered a normal component of the adult EEG awake. However, if the occipital alpha rhythm is absent, such a central theta rhythm may be normal, for such a condition is characteristic of physiological drowsiness. Because of these empirically determined facts, it is reasonable practice to begin the evaluation of a given EEG with specifications of the presence or absence of occipital alpha, and, if it is present, to characterize it in terms of the above features.

Frequency. The range of normal frequency for the occipital rhythm has been established on an empirical basis as 8 to 13 cycles per second for the adult.

Voltage. The voltage range is from 5 to 100 μV, but a detectable voltage at the scalp may not be present in a normal individual, a factor which relates more to the thickness and character of the scalp and skull than to the actual voltage at the cortex.

Locus. We specified occipital as the source of the particular rhythm under consideration. Locus is a prime consideration in evaluating a rhythm and its significance.

Four rhythms of similar (alpha) frequency and voltage are shown in Figs. 1–4. The first example is the bilaterally occurring *occipital* alpha of a normal adult in repose with eyes closed. The second example is the bilaterally occurring *frontal* alpha rhythm of an adult in a comatose state secondary to the ingestion of morphine.

The locus of these two bilateral alpha rhythms is the sole determinant of

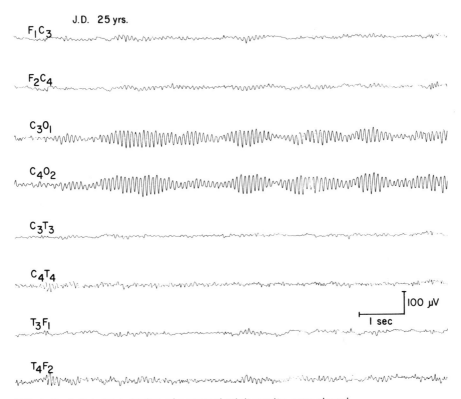

FIG. 1. Occipital alpha rhythm of a normal adult awake, eyes closed.

their differential significance. Their frequency, voltage, and wave form are similar, but the occipital rhythm signals normal wakefulness, the frontal rhythm a comatose state. Failure to recognize the importance of locus in determining the significance of a rhythm has led to some foolish mistakes in interpreting computerized data. Thus, patients undergoing surgery have been presumed to be awake on the basis of a spectral analysis that showed a maximum peak in the alpha frequency range, when in reality this activity was of frontal origin and characteristic of various anesthetic agents, including morphine and fluothane. The occipital region, the site of the dominant alpha rhythm awake, shows no sustained activity in the alpha range during anesthesia with these agents.

Interestingly, the ideal level of surgical anesthesia with these agents is characterized by sustained bifrontal alpha activity similar in frequency to the occipital alpha rhythm that the same patient showed awake. The anesthetic state is characterized by an anterior shift of the alpha rhythm.

Another type of a bilateral frontal alpha rhythm is not shown. This rhythm, in the context of sleep, has the opposite significance to that of the frontal alpha induced by certain anesthetic and hypnotic drugs. It appears transiently with spontaneous or evoked arousal in an adult who has been in any stage of sleep except Stage 1. Thus, the state of alertness as well as the site of a rhythm determine its significance.

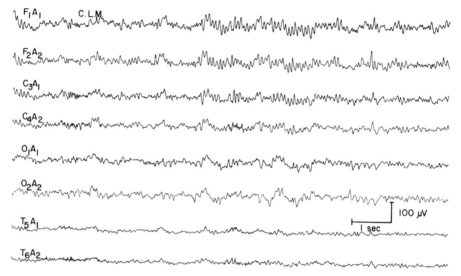

FIG. 2. Frontal dominant rhythmic activity of alpha frequency in a comatose patient following morphine administration.

The third example (Fig. 3) is a unilateral alpha rhythm arising focally in the right posterior-temporal region. Except for its unilateral focal occurrence, the rhythm is indistinguishable from the other three examples. This rhythm of alpha frequency is an electrographic manifestation of a clinical seizure in an infant at an age at which no sustained alpha rhythms are normally present.

Another example of an abnormal alpha frequency rhythm, is not illustrated. This one, a bilateral electrographic sign of epileptic discharge in the brain, has been reported by Gastaut. This rhythm is abnormal on the basis of its peak voltage and the paroxysmal character of its occurrence. Wave form, frequency, and even the chief locus of its appearance (occipital) are "normal."

The fourth example shown (Fig. 4) is a bilateral alpha rhythm which differs from the others in its wave form and its locus. This is the so-called mu

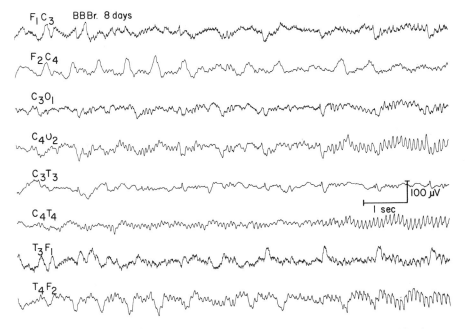

FIG. 3. Onset of rhythmic 10.5 cps activity in the right temporal and occipital leads occurring as part of a seizure in an infant of 8 days. This type of alpha rhythmic activity is usually seen in association with clinical seizures which are predominantly autonomic in character.

rhythm, a normal rhythm with activity of alpha frequency which is central in origin and which is distinguished by the initial, sharp, surface-negative phase of its wave form. Also, unlike the occipital alpha rhythm which is *bilaterally* reactive (blocks) to eye opening, the mu rhythm blocks *unilaterally* to motor activity of the extremities of the opposite side (e.g., opening and closing the hand).

The predominant alpha rhythm of the EEG of the normal adult is occipital in location, but there are other alpha generators which may be detected in scalp records in the central and temporal regions. As we have shown for the central alpha rhythm, each of these has different and specific characteristics.

Wave Form. The occipital alpha rhythm has a wave form approximating a sinusoid. Normal variation of this wave form includes so-called doubling or alpha variants.

Interhemispheric Coherence. The degree of congruence of the various parameters of the activity on the two sides is called interhemispheric coherence. The occipital alpha rhythm should have identical frequency characteristics on both sides. (Some authorities believe that a difference of 1

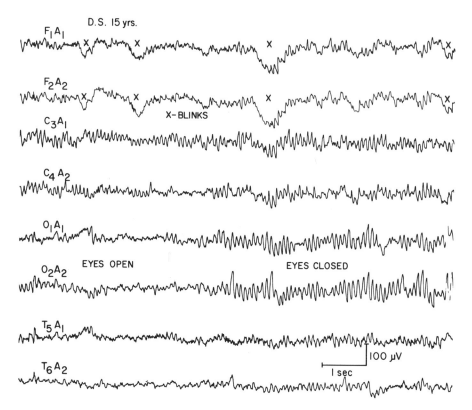

FIG. 4. Note the continuous mu-type alpha rhythm in the central leads with eyes open and closed. Note that the occipital alpha rhythm is blocked with eyes open. The wave form of the central mu rhythm is sharper than the occipital alpha rhythm.

cycle per second is acceptable.) However, some asymmetry of voltage is a characteristic of the normal brain, the voltage usually being lower on the side of the dominant hemisphere. Permissible voltage asymmetry is presently considered to be 50% if the low side is the dominant hemisphere, and 10% if the nondominant hemisphere is the low side.

Wave form should be similar on the two sides, although differences may sometimes be produced by the interference with other frequencies, e.g., fast, which may be present on the one side only.

The degree of synchrony of the activity of the two sides may be considered in terms of individual waves or of wave trains.

The occipital alpha rhythm tends to show good synchronization between sides not only of individual waves but of wave-train envelopes.

Character of Wave Occurrence. The name *alpha rhythm* specifies the manner of occurrence of the wave elements of this activity. The name is used (probably inappropriately) to refer to a train of waves of similar wavelength and wave form.

Such a wave train may be further characterized in terms of its persistence as constant or intermittent. If intermittent and of moderate voltage, it may be said to occur in "runs" or "bursts"; if it occurs with a sudden marked increase in voltage over the background activity, it may be referred to as a paroxysm (see Voltage Regulation, below).

In addition to a train or rhythm, the wave elements of the EEG may occur in "random" fashion.

Frequency Regulation. Frequency regulation is a measure of the consistency of wavelength in a given wave train. The occipital alpha rhythm tends to show good frequency regulation, the variation usually being less than ±0.5 cycle per second. This regulation tends to break down with increasing age and the corresponding development of cerebrovascular insufficiency (Sulg, 1969). Poor frequency regulation has been characterized by some electroencephalographers as a "pace dysrhythmia," and abnormal conditions other than vascular insufficiency may produce a breakdown of regulation.

Voltage Regulation. The voltage of the occipital alpha rhythm usually waxes and wanes within a relatively smooth envelope. Poor voltage regulation may be associated with the same conditions that produce poor frequency regulation.

Reactivity. The occipital alpha rhythm is reactive to eye opening and eye closing. It is more continuous or more "abundant" when the eyes are closed. Eye opening blocks the rhythm, but some return of activity may occur if the eyes remain open for more than a few seconds. The rhythm is also blocked by mental concentration and by alerting stimuli.

The steps of visual analysis which I have applied to the normal occipital alpha rhythm are applicable to any EEG activity and are the basis for determining the type and degree of an existing abnormality. The significance of a given wave or group of waves is generally determined by the interrelationship of two or more of the parameters described above.

VISUAL ANALYSIS AND THE DETERMINATION OF ABNORMALITY

Frequency/Voltage Ratio

The frequency/voltage ratio is an important factor of clinical evaluation. In general, whether a wave or wave train is of high or low voltage is assessed in terms of the wavelength of the activity, partly as a consequence of the manner in which the two factors generally are related in the EEG and partly because very slow waves are generally considered to be the product of the synchronized activity of many neurons. The more neurons, the greater the "expected" voltage. In terms of everyday EEG experience, slow waves in sleep are seen with amplitudes close to 0.5 mV. Beta activity is rarely seen with amplitudes much above 75 mV. Thus, the electroencephalograph considers a 50-μV wave with a wavelength of 1 sec as low voltage, whereas 35 cycle-per-second activity at 50 μV is regarded as "large" amplitude.

Another aspect of visual analysis is the relationship between the voltage of a given electrical event and the voltage of the background activity. A tacit assumption is made that the voltage of the alpha, for example, is largely a reflection of the attenuating characteristics of the tissues separating the brain and the electrode and an electrical event. For example, a random slow wave is rated as high or low voltage in terms of the voltage of the background.

Locus

The significance of the locus of an electrical event has been considered in some detail in the preceding analysis of alpha activity. The concept applies to all EEG phenomena, but it is essential to recognize that other parameters may influence the significance of the locus. To illustrate, Fig. 5 shows a sample of a tracing in which there are recurrent sharp-wave transients in the central region on the left side only. The configuration and temporal course of these transients are such that they could qualify within the limitations of visual analysis as the normal vertex transients of Stages 2 and 3 sleep, in which case their absence on the right side would indicate a destructive or depressive lesion of the *right* hemisphere. On the other hand, if the patient were awake, in Stage 1 sleep, or comatose, such sharp waves would indicate a lesion of the *left* hemisphere, because under such circumstances they signal an entirely different brain mechanism — an irritative focal pathological process involving the cortex (PLEDS or periodic lateralized epileptic discharge).

The similarity of these two entirely different phenomena is illustrated by comparison of Fig. 5 with Fig. 6. Figure 6 is a sample of tracing from a patient in Stage 2 sleep who had had a hemispherectomy; a subdural hematoma could produce a similar feature. Figure 5 is an example of PLEDS, a focal epileptic discharge arising from the left central region in a patient with an ischemic focal cortical lesion.

Wave Form

The evaluation of wave form to determine abnormality is probably the most complex problem encountered in the automatic analysis of the EEG, perhaps because it is most difficult for the electroencephalographer to specify for computer analysis what steps he takes in the visual analysis of a wave form. A given electrical event must be distinguished as normal, abnormal, or artifact, and, as demonstrated above, the state of wakefulness of the patient may be a prime determinant of whether a particular event is normal or abnormal.

In terms of wave form itself, a good rule of thumb is that in the waking state all activity should be of relatively simple wave form: the more complex the form and the sharper or more square-topped the configuration, the less likely the activity is to be a normal brain wave. To distinguish automatically between abnormal electrical events of cerebral origin and artifacts is much more complex, and because the clinical electroencephalographer finds it difficult to specify the factors by which he makes his discriminations, he offers little help. This is particularly true of the electrograms of newborn infants, in which abnormal electrical phenomena of the immature brain may

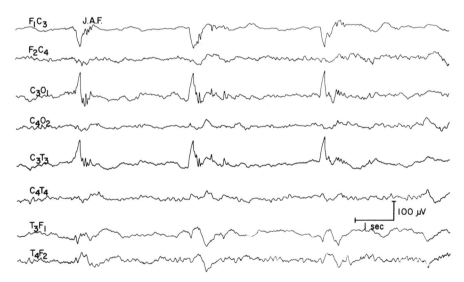

FIG. 5. Sharp waves followed by a brief train of fast waves in the left central region. This is the so-called periodic lateralized epileptic discharge (PLEDS). Recurrent focal, clinical, and electrographic seizures were recorded from the left central region. Compare with Fig. 6.

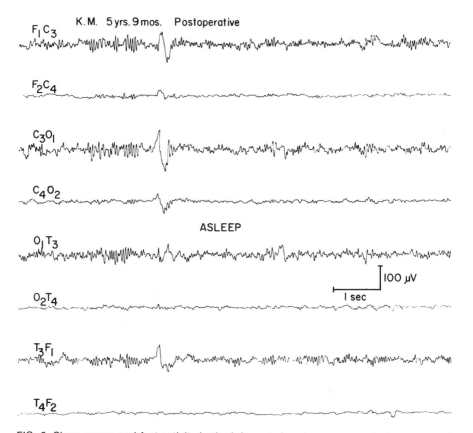

FIG. 6. Sharp waves and fast activity in the left central region are normal phenomena of Stage II sleep. They are depressed or absent from the right side because the patient had a right hemispherectomy.

look like artifacts, and the patient artifacts unique to this period of life (e.g., hiccoughing, sucking) simulate abnormal brain potentials (see Figs. 7 and 8). Even the discrimination between spikes of cerebral origin and various artifactual spikes is a human-computer process of some complexity. It is, in fact, a process not entirely mastered by many clinical electroencephalographers.

Maulsby has attempted with some success to provide guidelines for distinguishing cerebral from artifactual spikes. These guidelines might serve as a beginning in the design of a computer program.

1. Every spikey-looking transient is an artifact until proved otherwise.
2. Spikes and sharp waves of cerebral origin always occupy a definable

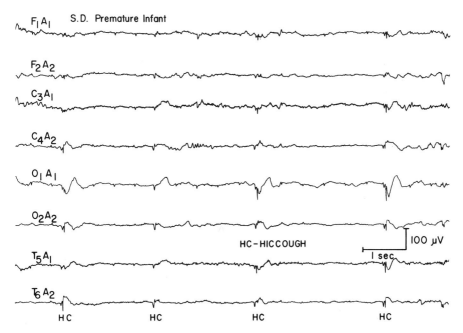

FIG. 7. Hiccough artifact in premature infant. Note similarity of wave form to the focal spike discharge of cerebral origin in Fig. 8.

electrical field at the scalp and should always be detected by at least one other adjacent electrode.

3. The initial component of clinically significant spikes and sharp waves is nearly always surface negative, or the sharpest or highest voltage component must be (surface) negative. (Exceptions: infant younger than 6 months, skull defect, or horizontal dipole.)

4. Most spike or sharp-wave discharges of clinical consequence are followed by a slow wave or a series of slow waves.

Interhemispheric Coherence

In the evaluation of interhemispheric congruence, age, state, locus, and the nature of the activity must each be considered. A reasonable basic rule in the adult is that normal activity is synchronous on the two sides and, with some special exceptions, bilaterally symmetrical.

The exceptions to bilateral voltage symmetry are as follows. (1) *The occipital alpha rhythm,* as outlined above. (2) *The central alpha or mu rhythm.* Marked asynchrony on the two sides is common. Consistent voltage

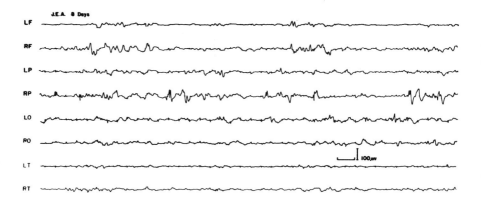

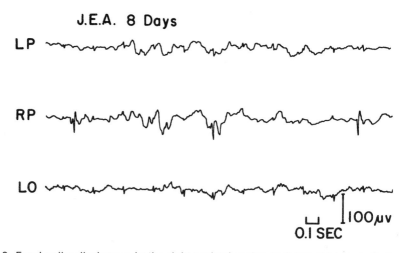

FIG. 8. Focal spike discharges in the right parietal region in 8-day-old infant. Surface-positive spike discharges rare in children and adults are not uncommon in the newborn. An enlargement of the spikes is shown at the bottom. Note the EKG artifact present. Recording uses homologous ear electrodes as reference. Compare with hiccough artifact in Fig. 7.

differences up to 50% are common, and laterality is not a consideration. (3) *Occipital positive theta.* This activity consists of runs of surface-positive sharp waves with a repetition rate of approximately 5 per second in the occipital region during light sleep. It is often asymmetric in homologous occipital leads on the two sides, and the degree of asymmetry is sometimes so marked in normal individuals as to suggest an abnormal focal discharge on one side—differentiation depends on repetition rate (5 per second), plus location, plus the major surface-positive wave element (a comparatively rare characteristic for an abnormal focal sharp-wave discharge).

Exceptions to Bilateral Synchrony

Sleep spindles (sigma) are asynchronous on the two sides from the time of their initial appearance at approximately 4 weeks until about the age of 1 year.

Consistent asynchrony of the spindles on the two sides is an abnormal finding in older children and adults. Asynchrony of the vertex sleep transients on the two sides is abnormal at any age and is a common finding in infants and young children with hydrocephalus.

In terms of automatic analysis, the phenomenon of voltage alternation would have to be taken into consideration by adequate time sampling. Voltage alternation is a phenomenon in which the spindles and vertex sharp-wave transients may appear in a given section of record to be asynchronous on the two sides but, in fact, is due to the voltage of these events, varying on the two sides. Thus, if in two successive bursts the voltage is low, first on one side then the other, asynchrony may be considered the reason: the occurrence of bilaterally synchronous spindle and vertex transients helps make the differentiation between the normal and the abnormal situation.

Bilateral synchrony is a characteristic of the mature EEG. In the premature infant there is no semblance of interhemispheric synchronization. With increasing age, increasing synchronization of the activity of the two sides takes place, first in the waking record, next in REM and transitional sleep, and last in deep sleep. Some asynchrony persists during the first month of life and is most marked in the temporal regions.

Character of Wave Occurrence

The manner in which the waves occur, either randomly or in a wave train continuously or intermittently, is an important aspect of evaluation of a child's EEG and, to a lesser extent, of adult records. Thus, the occurrence of random waves of 0.5-sec duration in the occipital leads bilaterally when intermixed with wave trains of 9 cycles per second might be a normal finding in a child of 8 years, but runs of rhythmic waves of the same frequency would be an abnormal finding.

The locus of an activity of a particular type also is a determining factor in its evaluation. Although random, moderate voltage, 0.5 per sec waves, mixed with alpha in the occipital region (Fig. 9) in a child may be normal, the same activity in the frontal region is abnormal.

Regulation. The character of the occurrence of waves is closely related in interpretation and regulation.

The sudden appearance of a frequency not previously present or minimally present with or without a sudden increase in voltage is a *paroxysmal* event and, with certain notable exceptions seen in sleep, is always an abnormal finding. Paroxysmal changes in voltage or frequency or both may involve single-wave elements as well as wave trains; a sudden transient involving a

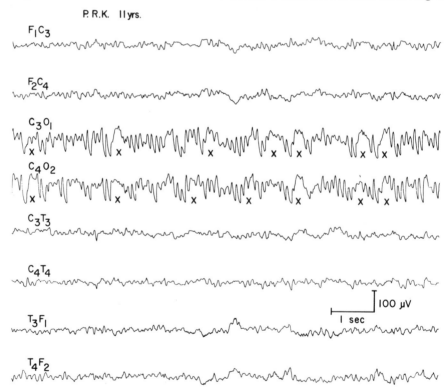

FIG. 9. This sample of the awake EEG of boy of 11 years shows the so-called "posterior slow waves of youth" in the occipital leads (cross marks). Bilateral random waves of this duration and voltage would be abnormal if found in any other region.

change of frequency or voltage or both (and often wave form) usually signifies abnormality.

Reactivity. Reactivity of an activity is used in diagnosis in various ways. For example, eye opening and closing may be used to determine if an occipital rhythmic slow-wave abnormality is a cortical or thalamocortical phenomenon: presumably, slow activity produced by a local cortical process would not block with eye opening, whereas a similar activity dependent upon thalamocortical mechanisms would block.

This aspect of EEG evaluation emphasizes the need for programmed control of situation and stimulus field.

Specific Electrographic Patterns. Specific electrographic patterns pose problems of pattern recognition of varying degrees of complexity, but the problems involved are probably no greater than for the other aspects of automatic analysis. Here again, interaction between expert electroencephalographer and computer scientist might facilitate the task by determining the minimal data necessary for recognition. Hypsarhythmia (Fig. 10) is probably

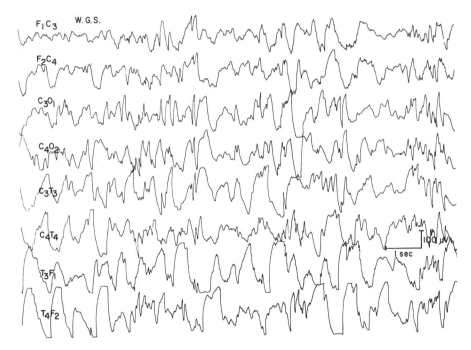

FIG. 10. Hypsarrhythmia. Note the very high voltage of the activity, the asynchrony and variable asymmetry between homologous leads, the spikes and sharp waves occurring at random in the various leads. It would be difficult to produce a template type of recognition system, but perhaps only a few sample criteria as mentioned in the text would discriminate this pattern in all its variations.

the most complex EEG pattern encountered. However, a highly discriminant recognition system might be based only on these simple criteria because of the unique character of the pattern. A basis for discrimination might be simply in terms of: (1) the very high voltage of the background rhythms; (2) spikes occurring asynchronously on two sides and in different sites; and (3) age. Several areas of EEG analysis provide more formidable tasks for automation; of these, the entire area of EEG application to the evaluation of premature and term infants probably constitutes the greatest difficulty.

CONCLUSIONS

The EEG probably presents the greatest complexities for signal processing and analysis of all medical laboratory tests. These complexities are a consequence of: (1) the multiplicity of the generators involved; (2) the variations that are consequent to changes in physiologic state; (3) the large number of wave patterns, normal and abnormal, which must be discriminated; (4) the close similarities between the electrical characteristics of artifacts and the physiological signals to be analyzed; and (5) the subtleties and multifactorial character of the process by which the clinical significance of the findings is derived.

Thus, if the automatic analysis and interpretation of clinical electroencephalography is possible, certainly that of other medically important biological signals cannot be far behind. Effective application of computer techniques to EEG should stimulate development of automation of other laboratory techniques and thus will serve a greater purpose in the large-scale delivery of effective health care.

APPENDIX

Analysis of EEG Record (Prepared by J. W. McSherry, M.D., Ph.D.)

Initial Information Input
1. Note the age and optimal state of consciousness of patient (e.g., alert, confused, lethargic, stuporous, or comatose)
2. Check technical characteristics of record (e.g., calibration, pen alignment, filters, symmetry run, and electrode resistance)
3. Enter run sequence

Run Sequence
1. Note electrode-channel array
2. Estimate state of consciousness in current 20-sec epoch (aroused, alert

but relaxed, drowsy, asleep (state I-IV and REM). Use certain well-described, key activities such as beta, occipital alpha, central sigma, and V waves, frontal sleep spindles, central mu, hypersynchronous drowsy 3 to 4 cps activity, occipital cone waves, and monophasic positive theta. If the state of consciousness cannot be specified, go to the "suspicious activity evaluation sequence" (SAES).

3. Are there any abnormalities of key activities, such as excessive assymetries, asynchronies, paroxysmal characteristics, poor regulation of frequency/amplitude, or other? If any key activity is abnormal, go to SAES.

4. Check the eight features of EEGs for consistency with the state of consciousness established. Is there anything else abnormal about the 20-sec epoch under investigation? If there are abnormalities, go to SAES.

5. Should a change have occurred during this 20-sec epoch that did not occur (e.g., alpha blocking with eye-opening, arousal from sleep with stimulation, or slowing with hyperventilation)? If a change was expected and did not occur, go to SAES.

6. Turn to next 20-sec epoch. If all the runs are complete, exit to Reporting. If there is a new run starting, go to step #1 of Run Sequence. If the current run is continuing, go to step #2 of Run Sequence.

Suspicious Activity Evaluation Sequence

1. If there are difficulites in defining state of consciousness, go to a special subroutine.
   (a) To evaluate at what point the state of consciousness became undefined—for instance, did the state change during the epoch, were there no key rhythms present, or were there predominantly features of one state but elements of another state?
   (b) To determine whether special activation procedures were occurring, such as stimulation of a sleeping patient, photic stimulation of a relaxed patient with eyes closed, or hyperventilation that might explain the events in (a).
   (c) To decide what should be done about (a) and (b)—increment suspicion index because no definite abnormality is seen but the record is still not right or note specific abnormality or ignore changes because either the abnormality has already been established previously or (b) explained (a) adequately and the tracing is still normal. Having completed (a)-(c), return to step in Run Sequence.

2. If the abnormality is in a key activity, go to a special subroutine.
   (a) To evaluate the nature of the abnormality (e.g., assymmetry of occipital alpha greater than 50%.

(b) To determine where the abnormality lies (e.g., one side depressed or the other side accentuated).
(c) To determine whether this is a consistent abnormality seen in previous epochs and runs or to be confirmed on subsequent epochs/runs (e.g., vertex sigma always depressed on the left side).
(d) To note if a compatible abnormality has been observed previously (e.g., consistent depression of all frequencies on the same side).
(e) To decide what should be done in view of (a)–(d) (e.g., in 6-month child, variable assymmetry and asynchrony of sigma would be ignored, consistent asynchrony would raise suspicion, and consistent assymmetry would constitute an abnormality).
3. If the abnormality is not in a key rhythm or definition of state, go to a special subroutine that identifies the abnormality as one of the following.
(a) One of a series of typical artifacts (e.g., electrode "pop").
(b) One of a set of typical abnormalities of cerebral function (e.g., frontal dominant, generalized 3/sec spike-and-wave).
(c) A focal or generalized abnormality consisting of specified frequencies, characterized by a certain onset/offset pattern and demonstrating specific reactivity characteristics.
The subroutine makes a decision on what to do about (a), (b), or (c). Artifact reduces confidence index on 20-sec epoch under study, recognized abnormality of cerebral origin enters abnormality in memory, and unclassified abnormality (most subjective aspect of reading EEGs) is judged to be probably artifact or probably cerebral in origin. In any case, events classified as (c) need confirmation in other epochs and runs and also in neighboring leads.

Reporting
1. Note terminal technical characteristics.
2. If the record is clearly normal, dictate.
3. If the record is abnormal but well defined (e.g., the only abnormality is bitemporal theta), dictate.
4. If the record is abnormal or apparently normal but the suspicion index is high, reread the record with closer attention to detail to confirm the abnormal or normal nature of the record. If after repeat reading there is still a high suspicion index, report the major finding with qualifiers (e.g., "there was some central slow but the patient appeared to be drowsy throughout the recording casting doubt on the diagnostic significance of this finding" or "borderline normal because of scattered fusing and a poorly regulated alpha."

5. If the EEG shows no specific abnormality but the confidence index is low because of artifact, reread the EEG excluding artifacts and decide if there is enough clean EEG on which to base a decision. Report it appropriately "EEG normal," or request a repeat examination for further evaluation.

DISCUSSION

Walter suggested that there are two approaches to EEG automation: (1) to define the perception and activities of an electroencephalographer when he interprets an EEG, and to program a machine to execute these functions; and (2) to apply pattern recognition methods developed in other fields to define the features that differentiate between EEGs belonging to different categories, without reference to techniques previously developed in clinical EEG practice. In other words, we must decide whether we should make a detailed imitation of what the electroencephalographer does, or let techniques developed in dead sciences govern what we do in live sciences. Walter then reported some general considerations regarding the types of discriminatory technique that can be applied to EEG diagnosis. Mathematical discriminatory methods are available which can be used to classify EEGs into different categories, and these could be applied without reference to clinical correlates. However, such a procedure could result in the classification of EEGs into groups which might have no clinical diagnostic relevance. Thus, although discrimination techniques that do not take clinical data into account may be applied to the research problem of developing better EEG descriptors, it seems probable that clinical correlative information will have to be used in developing a practical automated EEG system.

Kaiser raised the question of how long a segment of EEG record was needed for clinical diagnostic purposes, and there was general agreement that this would depend on the clinical situation, and that some automatically adaptive process which would sequence the EEG examination according to the characteristics of incoming information would be desirable. Thus the procedure and recording time would be different for a normal adult as compared, for example, with an abnormal child.

Discussion then turned to the potential usefulness of functionally limited EEG automation systems which do not provide comprehensive automation of the entire process from detection of the EEG signal to the production of an evaluation of the clinical significance of the findings. It was noted that quantitative techniques which result in data compression without loss of clinically significant information regarding EEG variability, or which perform simple pattern recognition and quantification functions, can reduce the time that must be spent by highly skilled personnel in EEG evaluation and are therefore economically worthwhile. Furthermore, these techniques can increase substantially the reliability of the EEG diagnostic process.

Petersén mentioned the difficulty of communicating the EEG findings to the clinician and pointed out that the same electrical findings might have different diagnostic significance in different clinical situations. Kellaway commented that a means of identifying automatically a normal EEG would be of great practical value, since 33.6% of the EEGs recorded in the Methodist Hospital laboratory, Houston, are classified as normal. However, an "electrically normal" EEG may be associated with brainstem dysfunction, and so it would seem that any fully automatic computer system must be able to use clinical as well as EEG information in formulating a diagnostic output.

In closing the discussion, Kellaway suggested that the process of automating clinical EEG would prove to be a step-by-step process, with the precision and economy of the diagnostic process increasing at each stage.

REFERENCES

Faure, J. (1950a): A une approche bio-électrique des émotions. *Journal de Physiologie,* 42:589–590.

Faure, J. (1950b): Methode d'évocation de potentials bio-electriques cérébraux par l'image chez le névropathe. *Journal de Medecine de Bordeaux et du Sud-Ouest,* 127:810–813.

Garsche, R. (1956): Die B-Aktivität im EEG des Kindes. *Zeitschrift für Kinderheilkunde,* 78:441–457.

Lairy, G. C. (1956): L'organisation de l'électroencephalogramme normale et pathologique. *Revue Neurologique,* 94:749–801.

Maulsby, R. L. (1971): An illustration of emotionally evoked theta rhythm in infancy: Hedonic hypersynchrony. *Electroencephalography and Clinical Neurophysiology,* 31:157–165.

Melin, K. A. (1953): The development of the electrical activity of the brain and its changes under pathological conditions. *Schweizer Archiv für Neurologie und Psychiatrie,* 71:217–223.

Sulg, I. A. (1969): The quantitated EEG as a measure of brain dysfunction. (*Academical thesis*). *Scandinavian Journal of Clinical and Laboratory Investigation,* 23, Suppl., 155 p.

Walter, W. G. (1950): Normal rhythms – Their development, distribution and significance. *In:* D. Hill and G. Parr (eds.), *Electroencephalography: A Symposium on Its Various Aspects.* Macmillan, New York, pp. 203–212.

Automation of Clinical Electroencephalography.
Edited by P. Kellaway and I. Petersén.
Raven Press, New York © 1973.

Need and Implementation of Centers for Automatic Analysis and Automatic Interpretation of Clinical EEG

I. Petersén, E. Kaiser and R. Magnusson

Department of Clinical Neurophysiology, Sahlgren Hospital, and Division of Applied Electronics, Chalmers University of Technology, Göteborg, Sweden, and the Kaiser Laboratory, Copenhagen, Denmark

In addition to the enormous amount of data contained in even a standard clinical recording, a striking feature of the human EEG is the considerable range of biological variation. Among the many parameters with which the EEG has been found to change are age, degree of alertness or sleep, sex, respiration and cerebral metabolism. The EEG is also influenced by a number of evocative procedures often employed in clinical EEG, *e.g.,* hyperventilation and photic stimulation. The way in which the EEG is affected by these parameters and procedures is, furthermore, modified by various diseases and injuries. Inter-individual differences are found not only in the EEG itself, but also in the sensitivity and mode of response to several of the factors mentioned above.

The accumulation and variability of data in an EEG recording render objective evaluation procedures highly desirable. This need is evident even when a number of recordings from a single patient are to be compared, and is, of course, still more pronounced when signals from different groups of patients or controls are handled. In view of this need, the several methods for automatic analysis of EEG developed in recent years become of considerable interest. Among these methods, the following, perhaps, are particularly relevant:

measurement of the amplitude distribution (Drohocki, 1939);

25

measurement of the duration distribution (duration being defined as the time interval between two successive zero crossings); (Stein, Goodwin and Garvin, 1949; Young, 1954);

pattern recognition, based on some combination of the two previous methods (Lonsdale, 1952; Kaiser and Sem-Jacobsen, 1962; Cohn, Leader, Weihrer and Caceres, 1967; Kaiser, Magnusson and Petersen, 1970),

spectrum analysis by means of narrow-band filters (Walter, 1943; Baldock and Walter, 1946; Kaiser and Petersén, 1966),

spectrum analysis by means of wide-band filters (Grass and Gibbs, 1938; Kozhevnikov, 1954; Kaiser, Petersén, Selldén and Kagawa, 1964);

spectrum analysis by means of the Fast Fourier Transform (Walter, 1963; Dumermuth and Flühler, 1967),

spectrum analysis according to Zetterberg (1968);

correlation analysis (Wiener, 1930, 1953; Brazier and Casby, 1952; Brazier and Barlow, 1956; Kaiser and Petersen, 1965; Kaiser, Magnusson and Petersén, 1969),

spectral moment analysis (Hjort, 1970); and

analysis of averaged evoked potentials (Dawson, 1947, 1954).

To a varying extent, these methods have been applied in clinical EEG research. To our knowledge they have not yet, however, been used to supplement the conventional evaluation of EEGs in clinical practice. There are several reasons for this delay in the application of the methods to the clinical diagnostic procedure. One reason is that many of the methods, although automatic, are quite time consuming. Another reason is the lack of information on mean values, dispersions and other statistical measures of the relevant EEG parameters of normal individuals and of patients with various diseases or injuries. In fact, there has even been a lack of a statistically sufficient number of EEG recordings from carefully selected and defined groups of normal subjects, and thus a *generally* insufficient knowledge of the EEG of normals, which in turn has imposed limitations on the correct classification of EEG findings in patients.

In the last few years very rapid analyses of the EEG have become possible owing to the development of high-speed specialized analyzers and computers. Furthermore, good-sized collections of EEG signals from subjects carefully selected with regard to clinical normality have been recorded on tape and are thus available for various kinds of visual and automatic analysis. Two main obstacles to the application in clinical EEG practice of automatic analysis have thus been removed. In our opinion, there are good reasons to expect that in the near future these methods will have a considerable impact on the description and evaluation of clinical

EEG. This impact will most probably concern not only the objectiveness of the parameter estimation but also the very *interpretation, i.e.,* the final diagnostic classification, of the individual EEG. In view of the instrumentation cost involved, it is reasonable to expect that the data processing will be performed at central laboratories serving quite large regions, and that the individual EEGs will be telemetered from peripheral standard-size laboratories to the "EEG Center." It is obvious that this type of organization will also provide various possibilities of rationalization, such as relieving the highly skilled EEG experts of much of the dull part of EEG reading and a general reduction of manpower involved.

The creation of EEG Centers of the type outlined above clearly requires very close cooperation between medical EEG experts and engineering experts in the fields of signal analysis, applied electronics and computer programming. The various methods of automatic analysis must be tested and compared with respect to their ability to resolve the pertinent EEG parameters, and with respect to the correlation of these parameters to clinical symptoms and signs. It should be stressed that the indispensable first step in this investigation is the determination of the parameter limits of EEGs from normal individuals. Once the optimal method or combination of methods has been found, the means of satisfying the need for increased objectiveness in EEG evaluation are available. The transmission of EEG recordings from peripheral laboratories to the EEG Center requires the development of telephone-line — or possibly wireless — telemetry systems capable of handling at least eight EEG channels and also information on parameters such as heart frequency and eye movements. The size of a particular EEG Center and of the region it serves will probably to a very great extent be determined by the technical and economical development of electronic computers.

The general concept of an EEG Center outlined above has, in fact, for nearly a decade formed one of the main themes in the EEG research program of the Neuronics Group constituted by the authors and their collaborators. It is also interesting to note that in 1970 a national committee was appointed by the Swedish Board for Technical Development, the Swedish Medical Research Council, and the Swedish Institute for Hospital Planning and Rationalization, with the object of coordinating research and development in the fields of automatic EEG analysis, including the creation of EEG Centers.

DISCUSSION

Frost asked Petersén to comment on what he considered to be the first step in practical automation of the EEG. Petersén replied that the first step would be to compare different methods of spectral analysis to try to determine which method, or combination of methods, would be best for describing the EEG. This approach would involve collecting and analyzing EEGs from normal subjects and from assorted groups of patients, and work on this stage of the project has begun.

REFERENCES

Baldock, G. R., and Walter, W. G. (1946): A new electronic analyzer. *Electronic Engineering*, 18:339–342.

Brazier, M. A. B., and Barlow, J. S. (1956): Some applications of correlation analysis to clinical problems in electroencephalography. *Electroencephalography and Clinical Neurophysiology*, 8:325–331.

Brazier, M. A. B., and Casby, J. U. (1952): Crosscorrelation and autocorrelation studies of electroencephalographic potentials. *Electroencephalography and Clinical Neurophysiology*, 4:201–211.

Cohn, R., Leader, H. S., Weihrer, A. L., and Caceres, C. A. (1967): Computer mensuration and interpretation of the human electroencephalogram (EEG). *Digest 7th International Conference on Medical and Biological Engineering*, Stockholm, p. 265.

Dawson, G. D. (1947): Cerebral responses to electrical stimulation of peripheral nerve in man. *Journal of Neurology, Neurosurgery and Psychiatry*, 10:134–140.

Dawson, G. D. (1954): A summation technique for the detection of small evoked potentials. *Electroencephalography and Clinical Neurophysiology*, 6:65–84.

Drohocki, Z. (1939): Elektrospektrographie des Gehirns. *Klinische Wochenschrift*, 18:536–538.

Dumermuth, G., and Flühler, H. (1967): Some modern aspects in numerical spectrum analysis of multichannel electroencephalographic data. *Medical and Biological Engineering*, 5:319–331.

Grass, A. M., and Gibbs, F. A. (1938): Fourier transform of the electroencephalogram. *Journal of Neurophysiology*, 1:521–526.

Hjort, B. (1970): EEG analysis based on time domain properties. *Electroencephalography and Clinical Neurophysiology*, 29:306–310.

Kaiser, E., Magnusson, R., and Petersén, I. (1969): Cross echo correlation. *Proceedings of the 8th International Conference on Medical and Biological Engineering*, Chicago, pp. 3–12.

Kaiser, E., Magnusson, R., and Petersén, I. (1970): A sixteen-channel wave-pattern digitizer. *Proceedings of the 1st Nordic Meeting on Medical and Biological Engineering*, Helsingfors, pp. 128–130.

Kaiser, E., and Petersén, I. (1965): A new method for detecting rhythmic activity in time series. *Communications of the 6th International Congress of Electroencephalography and Clinical Neurophysiology*, pp. 535–537.

Kaiser, E., and Petersén, I. (1966): Automatic analysis in EEG. *Acta Neurologica Scandinavica*, 42: Suppl. 22.

Kaiser, E., Petersen, I., Selldén, U., and Kagawa, N. (1964): EEG data representation in broad-band frequency analysis. *Electroencephalography and Clinical Neurophysiology*, 17:76–80.

Kaiser, E., and Sem-Jacobsen, C. W. (1962): "Yes-no" data reduction in EEG automatic pattern recognition. *Electroencephalography and Clinical Neurophysiology*, 14:955.

Kozhevnikov, V. A. (1954): A method of automatic analysis of biopotentials (an electronic analyzer of the biopotentials of the brain). *Fiziologicheskiu Zhurnal S.S.S.R.*, 40:487–492.

Lonsdale, M. E. (1952): Development of a statistical analyzer for random waveforms. State University of Iowa Doctoral Dissertation Series, 4084.

Stein, S. N., Goodwin, C. W., and Garvin, A. (1949): A brain wave correlator and preliminary studies. *Transactions of the American Neurological Association*, 74:196–199.

Walter, D. O. (1963): Spectral analysis for electroencephalograms: Mathematical determination of neurophysiological relationships from records of limited duration. *Experimental Neurology*, 8:155–181.

Walter, W. G. (1943): An automatic low frequency analyzer. *Electronic Engineering*, 16:9–13.

Wiener, N. (1930): Generalized harmonic analysis. *Acta Mathematica*, 55:117–257.

Wiener, N. (1953): Discussion in EEG technics. *Electroencephalography and Clinical Neurophysiology*, Suppl. 4:41–44.

Young, F. M. (1954): Probability distribution of zero-crossing intervals. *Massachusetts Institute of Technology Acoustics Laboratory Quarterly Progress Report No. 3.*

Zetterberg, L. H. (1968): Estimation of parameters for a linear difference equation with application to EEG analysis. Report 18, *Teletransmissionsteori KTH and Mathematical Biosciences*, 5:227–275.

Automation of Clinical Electroencephalography.
Edited by P. Kellaway and I. Petersén.
Raven Press, New York © 1973.

A Sleep-Analysis System as a Model of Automation of Clinical Electroencephalography

James D. Frost, Jr.

Department of Neurophysiology, The Methodist Hospital, and Baylor College of Medicine, Houston, Texas 77025

The conference participants have discussed in some detail a number of methodologies for accomplishing analysis of EEG activity, and although these statistical, mathematical, and electronic techniques represent an essential aspect of the problem at hand, it is important not to lose sight of nor to forget the significance of the other two equally important aspects of clinical EEG automation; data acquisition and presentation, or reporting the results. We must consider the entire system of acquisition, analysis, and display techniques if we ever hope to attain automated electroencephalography.

A brief discussion of the sleep-monitoring system currently under development for use in the Skylab series of manned space flights will illustrate the point. Although sleep analysis is certainly a very restricted area of EEG, the problems we have encountered and the approach to their solutions can serve as a rudimentary, if incomplete, model of a more general EEG automation system.

The system is composed of a recording cap with seven electrodes for two EEG and one EOG channels; a preamplifier including a dual-axis accelerometer for detection of head motion; a control unit contining final amplification and electrode testing circuitry as well as an analog tape recorder; an analysis section accepting the EEG, EOG, and head motion signals and providing an output indication of sleep stage; and the display console.

Figure 1 shows a prototype version of the sleep-monitoring apparatus. The items in the lower portion, concerned with acquisition and analysis, are located onboard the spacecraft; the data-display console, shown in the upper portion, is located on the ground to receive the telemetered results.

The recording cap with electrolyte-saturated sponge sensors acquires EEG and EOG signals from the subject during sleep periods. The signals are amplified initially by a small preamplifier unit (which also contains an accelerometer for head-motion detection) attached to the cap. Signals are then led to the control-panel unit for final amplification, and the raw data are preserved on analog tape. The analysis unit processes signals online, providing the telemetry system an output indicative of the sleep stage. This output is transmitted to the ground-based display console which produces a graph of sleep stage versus time and accumulates a record of the amount of time spent in each sleep stage.

Acquisition of EEG and EOG signals during space flight poses numerous

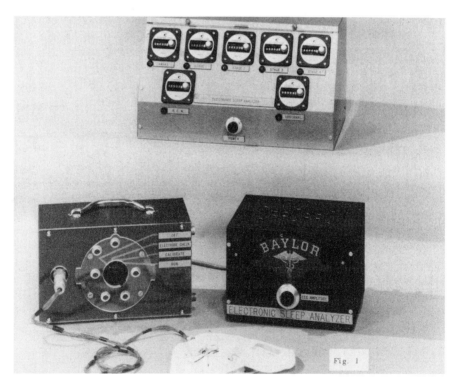

FIG. 1. View of total system.

problems, some similar to those encountered in routine clinical EEG. Because of the subject's inaccessibility, however, we have been forced to reconsider many of the routine solutions. Consequently, we have in effect automated a number of the procedures ordinarily performed by an EEG technician, and some of these special-purpose technical innovations may eventually be adapted to the analogous problems in clinical EEG and may result in time and cost savings.

Almost all situations involving EEG recording outside the laboratory entail problems associated with electrodes. Preparation time must be minimized — it is not feasible to allot 15–20 min before each recording session to attach and check out electrodes as we do in the clinical lab. Technical personnel are not available, and so the astronaut himself or another member of the crew must apply the electrodes. Finally, conventional electrodes are not reliable enough; if they fall off during a sleep period, there is usually no chance to reapply them.

The recording cap displayed in Fig. 2 has slowly and painfully evolved over the last several years. It utilizes the sponge-type electrode concept which originated in Dr. Adey's laboratory several years ago (Adey, Winters, Kado, and De Lucchi, 1963; Kado, Adey, and Zweizig, 1964; Kado and Adey, 1968; Hanley, Zweizig, Kado, Adey, and Rovner, 1969; Hanley, Adey, Zweizig, and Kado, 1971). The present configuration and sensor construction have been changed considerably to meet the current requirements. In terms of automation, the most important new feature of this recording cap is that it is ready to use. Each sponge electrode affixed to the inside of the cap is prefilled with an electrolyte gel during manufacture.

A cross-section of the electrode (Fig. 3) shows the sponge portion, the conical shape of which facilitates penetration through the hair; the base of the cone makes contact with a conventional silver/silver chloride disc. After the sponge is affixed to the base, the entire electrode is covered with a thin, continuous coating of flexible vinyl plastic. Electrolyte is injected into the sponge through the top, and the top is sealed with vinyl. The cap may then be stored indefinitely until needed. At the time of intended use, the subject removes the cap from its storage bag and, as illustrated in Fig. 4, clips off the sealing tip of each electrode, thereby exposing the electrolyte-saturated sponge.

To illustrate the time-saving aspect of this acquisition system, below is a thumbnail sketch of the sequence followed in an actual recording situation.

The subject follows a simple procedure requiring 2 min or less to render the recording cap operational. He (1) removes the cap from its storage bag, (2) attaches the preamplifier to the vertex of the cap, (3) cuts off the sealing tabs from each electrode, (4) dons the cap, (5) tests the electrodes automati-

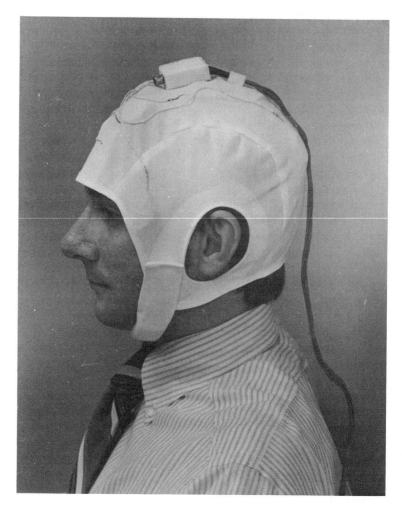

FIG. 2. Cap properly positioned on subject.

cally by turning the selector switch on the control panel to the "test" mode (if the interelectrode resistance is less than 100,000 ohms, a panel lamp corresponding to the appropriate cap electrode is illuminated), and (6) proceeds with recording by turning the selector switch to the "run" position.

The cap is disposable after use, thus eliminating the problems associated with storage of most electrodes. Since a cap may be packed in a very small container, it is feasible to take a supply sufficient for each planned recording session.

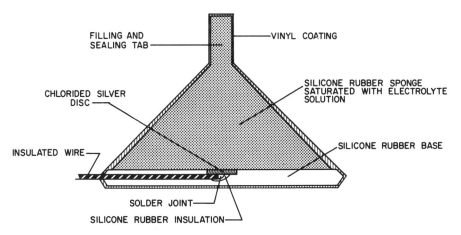

FIG. 3. Cross section of prefilled sponge electrode.

The data-analysis circuitry in this system has a well-defined task; it must constantly produce an output indicative of the subject's current sleep status. Consequently the output is restricted to seven levels, corresponding to the conditions of Awake, Stages 1–4 and REM of sleep as well as an Abnormal category which includes all conditions that do not fit into one of the other categories.

This unit is a hybrid device employing numerous analog and digital circuits, and although it is relatively simple, there is considerable interaction between the various sections. The attempt has been made in designing the device to achieve a true automation of sleep scoring; the circuitry incorporates basically the same criteria for distinguishing sleep stages visually from a graphic record.

In brief, the four major sections function as illustrated in the logic diagram shown in Fig. 5. The most basic analysis is accomplished in the EEG section, which operates as an amplitude-weighted frequency meter. Activity from a single central-to-occipital bipolar channel is processed to obtain an "analog of sleep" signal covering Stages 1–4. Operation of the EEG section is most easily visualized using a graphic example (Fig. 6). This circuitry recognizes three amplitude levels above baseline. One-hundred percent is set as a convenient but arbitrary level, and the others are determined with respect to the distance between it and the zero baseline of the EEG signal. The EEG gain does not have to be adjusted for each subject; the circuitry employs a fixed gain setting which is 19.0 μV peak equivalent to level 3, or 100%.

A train of pulses is produced, as indicated in the lower trace (Fig. 6), as the EEG signal crosses the various levels. A wave which crosses only level 1 results in no output; that is, it is assigned a value of zero. A deflection which crosses level 1 and level 2 in that order produces a negative pulse of unit size. Fluctuations about level 2 alone do not result in output pulses, nor do downward crosses. The train of negative pulses is consequently proportional to the *dominant* EEG frequency. If a wave crosses levels 1, 2, and 3, the usual negative pulse is produced as 1 and 2 are crossed, but a positive pulse of one-half the amplitude of the negative pulse occurs as the 3rd level is exceeded. This means that a large-amplitude wave has a value equivalent to one-half that of an intermediate-amplitude wave when the

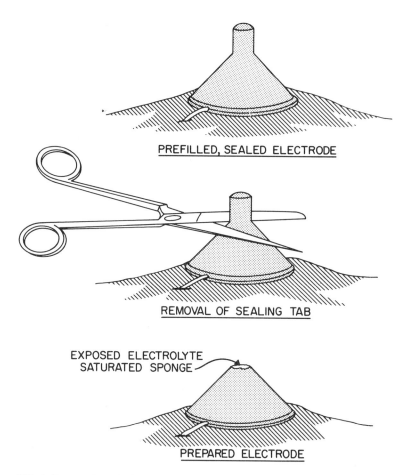

PREFILLED, SEALED ELECTRODE

REMOVAL OF SEALING TAB

EXPOSED ELECTROLYTE
SATURATED SPONGE

PREPARED ELECTRODE

FIG. 4. Preparation of electrode for use.

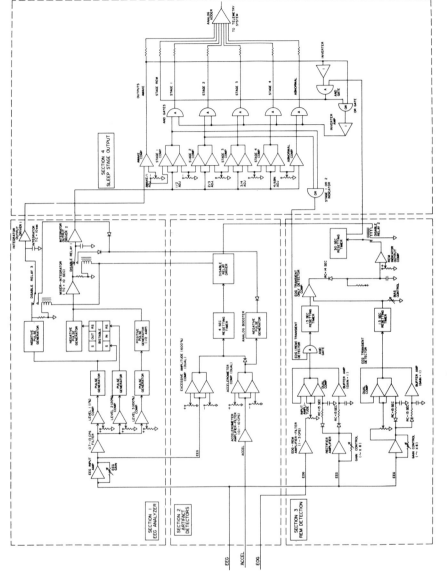

FIG. 5. Logic diagram of analysis circuitry.

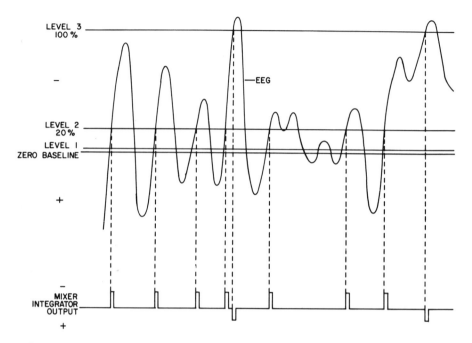

FIG. 6. EEG analysis scheme.

pulse train is integrated, whereas a small-amplitude wave has no value.

The Awake state is determined solely on the basis of dominant frequency. The level 1 comparator changes its output state each time the EEG crosses the 1% baseline level. The positive-going deflections drive the negative-pulse generator, which produces a constant amplitude and duration pulse each time the EEG crosses the baseline in a positive-going direction. The train of pulses from the negative-pulse generator is integrated with a 10-sec time constant. The output of this integrator (output driver 1 voltage level) is consequently proportional only to the dominant EEG frequency and is independent of amplitude.

The pulse train enters an RC integration circuit with a time constant of 10 sec, and this integrator's output is therefore a voltage level which is highest when the EEG signal is of high frequency and intermediate amplitude, such as when the subject is awake. This scheme takes advantage of the EEGs progressive decline in frequency and the progressive increase in amplitude during the transition from Awake to Stage 4 sleep.

This analog signal is therefore proportional to sleep stage on a scale extending from Awake at the high end to Stage 4 at the low end. It enters the analyzer's output stage where it is observed by a series of dual comparator circuits (Fig. 5, section 4), each set to detect a predetermined range of the analog signal which corresponds to a specific sleep stage. The analyzer output corresponding to the sleep stage is activated if the other criteria are met. No attempt is made in the EEG analysis scheme to separate Stage REM, and it will be classified as either Stage 1 or Stage 2, based solely on its EEG characteristics. Stage REM is, however, detected by the EOG analysis section (Fig. 5, section 3).

The basic problem here is detection of true REMs from the EOG signal while rejecting similar wave forms resulting from EEG transients, such as K-complexes, which also appear in the EOG channel. Amplified EOG activity enters the analyzer through a narrow bandpass analog filter which limits the response to the 1–3 Hz range. This response results in optimal but not perfect separation of true REMs from extraneous activity.

This filtered signal enters the EOG-transient detector, which indicates the occurrence of a transient form exceeding a positive or negative value equivalent to 250% of the average positive or negative peak voltage value of the EEG signal for the preceding 5 sec. This transient detection is accomplished by driving the upper and lower voltage reference inputs of a dual comparator circuit with the rectified and filtered positive and negative components, respectively, of the EEG amplifier output signal. The EOG enters the comparator common input, after appropriate attenuation, where it is continuously compared to the upper and lower reference values.

This circuit is effective in detecting REMs, as these events usually occur sporadically and arise abruptly from the background activity. Since the circuit detects an increase in amplitude compared to the average of the preceding 15 sec of EEG instead of utilizing fixed-voltage references, it is not necessary to readjust the sensitivity for individual differences in EEG amplitude. Similarly, a change in background activity level during the course of sleep causes the reference levels to reset automatically to appropriate relative values, thereby preventing false triggering.

Although the REM detector successfully recognizes most true REMs, it will also be triggered by certain EEG-transient events because of their similarity in wave form and frequency components. This problem is resolved by including an EEG-transient detector (Fig. 5, section 3) which operates in a manner similar to the EOG-transient detector, but in this case the EEG channel is the input to the comparator as well as the driving source for the references. Since true REMs are recorded only in the EOG channel, the final logic scheme prevents an output REM indication if a transient is detected by the EEG circuit within a time window extending from 1.4 sec before until 1.4 sec after the EOG event. In addition, a REM cannot be detected unless the EEG analysis section (Fig. 5, section 1) is in either Stage 1 or Stage 2, thereby preventing the eye movements associated with the Awake state from interfering.

If a true REM is detected in Stage 1 or 2, it activates a 30-sec timer which switches the final analyzer output to Stage REM. If a REM is detected at least once per 30 sec, the output will remain in Stage REM, otherwise it will revert back to the stage indicated by the EEG analysis section.

The final section of the analyzer (Fig. 5, section 2) is concerned with artifacts. Although the EEG and EOG acquisition methods have been designed to minimize the occurrence of artifactual signals, it has not yet been possible to eliminate them. This section prevents signals with a high probability of artifactual contamination from influencing the sleep stage determination systems; this is accomplished by disabling the EEG and EOG analysis sections during and for 4 sec following either of two events: (1) a period of excessive EEG amplitude as determined by an amplitude comparator set at a relative value of ±600% or, (2) a head movement resulting in an acceleration change of approximately 0.2 in either the vertical or lateral axis.

The first event, large EEG amplitude, is not likely to represent physiological activity and is most often a result of changing electrode contact potentials, such as when a subject rolls over in bed. Similarly, the presence of head motion indicates that an artifact is likely to occur because of changing electrode contact with the surroundings. When disabled, the analyzer simply maintains the current stage as determined by the EEG section, and incoming data have no influence.

The final output of the system's analysis portion is telemetered to the ground-based display console as a three-bit code sent at a rate of approximately one code per second.

The display console (see Fig. 1, upper portion) accepts the reconstituted sleep stage signal from the telemetry receiver and provides an easily readable record of the sleep characteristics. A panel lamp illuminates to indicate the current stage of sleep, and an associated cumulative time indicator records the total time spent in each sleep stage throughout the night. A graphic record is produced simultaneously (Fig. 7) which illustrates the progression of sleep stages during the recording period.

Some brief speculation may be entertained on the potential value of such a system in the clinical situation with which we are concerned today. In terms of the overall system, the first question is, "How well does it work?" This is not an easy question, and the answer can really be adequately conveyed only by actually using the system. One frequently used method is to look at plots of the results of human and machine scoring, and in general they appear quite similar. In other words, both come up with the same number of

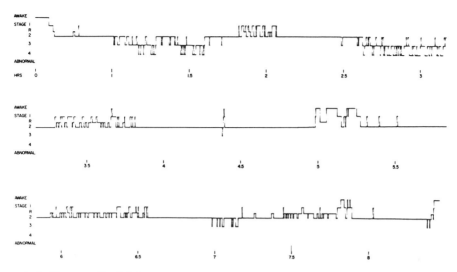

FIG. 7. Sleep profile (8 hr).

sleep cycles and roughly the same pattern. A more precise way is to express the absolute agreement between the two methods on an epoch-for-epoch basis; that is, of all the epochs scored by the human, what percentage was scored exactly the same by the analyzer? Looked at this way, the agreement is usually between 70 and 80%. The system is certainly adequate for a general screening of sleep patterns, and when comparing sleep from night to night under different circumstances, it is in many ways more consistent in its behavior than is a human scorer. On the other hand the machine is still not as good as the human in some areas, particularly the precise detection of REM periods.

The most significant lesson learned, largely the hard way, from developing this apparatus is the extreme importance of the data acquisition process and the related necessity for dealing specifically with artifacts. A human is an excellent artifact detector; he does it almost unconsciously. This trait makes him capable of dealing with his everyday environment and in fact makes him a good electroencephalographer. However, it makes him a poor computer programmer or analyzer builder. He constantly either tries to do the job for the machine by presorting the data, or he simply forgets that the artifact exists, or quite often he goes ahead and solves the problem with the assumption that someone else will provide clean data. If we are ever going to truly automate EEG, we must begin to deal with the problem right at the electrodes and follow it all the way through.

Another lesson to be learned is the considerable computational power which is easily available to the designer of such hybrid devices. It would require a fairly complex digital computer program to duplicate the functions of this relatively simple analyzer. This is not to suggest that the job of clinical automation can or should be done by hybrid devices alone, but we should begin serious attempts to utilize both approaches in an integrated way. The EEG machine itself is an analog computer of sorts, and there is no reason why it should not be considered as an important and *interactive* component of the system.

A final aspect of great importance in the clinical situation is the problem of data display. The designer of automated systems must learn to swallow his pride and show only the *answer,* not the intermediate data. To use the sleep system as an example, the preferred output format would be a multichannel graphic recording showing all the intermediate steps in the analysis process because these are interesting to the inventor, and they are more impressive in that they *prove* that the box is really doing something. However, no one else wants to see these things; all they want to know is the stage of sleep, no more. Consequently, the system must do just that whether the designer wants to or not. The same thing is true for all of clinical automation; the physician will never be impressed with a spectral plot, or a table of period counts, or a contour map, or any other intermediate step, no matter how essential it is to the overall process. We need always to carry the analysis beyond these points and to define the output in a simple way.

DISCUSSION

Walter and Larsen commented on the importance of excluding information due to artifact that may be mixed with an EEG signal. Maulsby observed that Frost has been highly successful in excluding movement artifact and that the type of logic circuitry that was used for this purpose might be applicable to several problems in EEG analysis and quantification.

In replying to a question from Walter, Frost mentioned that there is an hysteresis around each transition level between sleep stages. This is actually an automated version of what the human does; examination of ratings of sleep records provided by electroencephalographers has shown that once a record has been scored as being in a particular sleep stage, the human rater is more reluctant to change his scoring to an earlier stage than to a later stage.

In a reply to a question from Kaiser, Frost said that sampling the output of the analyzer every 10 sec, for example, for telemetry purposes, gives essentially the same output pattern as that obtained by continuous sampling.

Remond said that this technique of sleep analysis represented a real breakthrough in EEG. He asked what baseline was used in identifying zero-crossing points, how many EEG channels were provided in the electrode cap, and how much interference was encountered. Frost replied that the signals coming into the analyzer were first passed through an analog band-pass filter with 3 dB points at 0.7 and 13.0 Hz. The baseline is taken as being the zero output from this filter. There are two EEG channels, both central-to-occipital, and either of these can be used by the analyzer. If one channel should develop a fault, the analyzer can be switched manually to the other channel. The electrode resistances are usually in the 30 to 50 kΩ range, but interference is not a problem for two main reasons: (1) the pre-amplifier is mounted right on the head, thus shortening the leads; and (2) the bandpass filters heavily attenuate interference at line 60-Hz frequency.

REFERENCES

Adey, W. R., Winters, W., Kado, R. T., and De Lucchi, M. R. (1963): EEG in simulated stresses of space flight with special reference to the problems of vibration. *Electroencephalography and Clinical Neurophysiology*, 15:305–320.

Hanley, J., Adey, W. R., Zweizig, J. R., and Kado, R. T. (1971): EEG electrode amplifier harness. *Electroencephalography and Clinical Neurophysiology*, 30:147–150.

Hanley, J., Zweizig, J. R., Kado, R. T., Adey, W. R., and Rovner, L. D. (1969): Combined telephone and radiotelemetry of the EEG. *Electroencephalography and Clinical Neurophysiology*, 26:323–324.

Kado, R. T., and Adey, W. R. (1968): Electrode problems in central nervous system monitoring in performing subjects. *Annals of the New York Academy of Sciences*, 148:263–278.

Kado, R. T., Adey, W. R., and Zweizig, J. R. (1964): Electrode system for recording EEG from physically active subjects. *Proceedings of the 17th Annual Conference on Engineering in Medicine and Biology*, 5.

Automation of Clinical Electroencephalography.
Edited by P. Kellaway and I. Petersén.
Raven Press, New York © 1973.

Toward an EEG Screening Test: A Simple System for Analysis and Display of Clinical EEG Data

Robert L. Maulsby, Bernard Saltzberg and Leonard S. Lustick

Tulane University School of Medicine, 1430 Tulane Avenue, New Orleans, Louisiana 70112

In the past decade, many excellent methods of computer analysis of EEGs have been developed and shown to be of practical value, but there has been no serious attempt to apply these techniques to routine clinical testing. The rapidly increasing load of clinical EEGs and the relative scarcity of qualified electroencephalographers make it imperative that we begin to utilize automation and computer techniques in routine diagnostic work.

Approaches to this goal could take two different routes: (1) automation of the tasks of the electroencephalographer from analysis through interpretation, or (2) simplification of EEG data by computers to facilitate interpretation of EEGs by clinicians who are not electroencephalographers, in effect, creation of more interpreters. The latter of these two approaches is obviously easier and was adopted for this feasibility study, the goal of which is to develop a reliable, quantitative EEG screening test useful in the bulk of EEG referrals to help the clinician decide if a gross cerebral lesion or disturbance exists and what type of further testing is required (for instance, conventional EEG, brain scan, or roentgenographic studies).

This chapter describes and presents the results of initial tests of a simple method of reducing multi-channel EEG data into a one-page display which can be comprehended readily by physicians without specialty training in EEG.

45

METHODS

The three subjects for this study were two neurologically normal females, ages 24 and 33, and one patient, age 33, who had mild left hemiparesis of recent onset and an angiographically proved arteriovenous malformation of the right fronto-parietal cortex.

Eight conventional EEG disc electrodes were placed over International 10–20 System electrode sites to obtain the following eight-channel "bipolar" montage: $F_{p1}-C_3$, $F_{p2}-C_4$, C_3-O_1, C_4-O_2, O_1-T_3, O_2-T_4, T_3-F_{p1}, T_4-F_{p2}.

The EEG was recorded on a magnetic tape recorder (Ampex, Model FR-1300) at $3\frac{3}{4}$ ips simultaneously with production of a standard ink-writing oscillographic recording on a Grass model 7 Polygraph. The time constant was 0.4 sec with high-frequency cutoff (50% down at 75 Hz). A standard IRIG B time code was later painted on the tape to allow searching.

The test procedure consisted of several alternating periods of resting in two conditions — eyes open and eyes closed — for 30 to 60 sec each. Recordings on magnetic tape were reproduced later on an ink-writer along with a slow BCD translation of the time code for visual selection of samples to be analyzed by the computer. Ten-sec epochs relatively free of artifacts (particularly eye-movement artifacts) were selected for each condition (eyes open and eyes closed) in each subject's record.

The selected epochs of each record were then reproduced through another set of differential DC amplifiers (Offner, Type R) in order to gain secondary derivations simulating referential recordings as illustrated in Fig. 1.

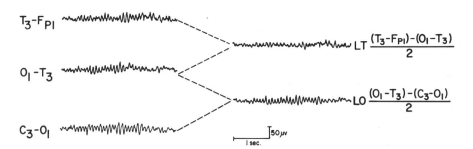

FIG. 1. Illustration of secondary derivations used for analysis. The primary derivations on the left are bipolar recordings which "mix" the rhythms from the active sites with respect to voltage. Detection of "phase reversals" must be used to determine where a given wave or rhythm arises. The secondary derivations on the right accomplish this to some extent by emphasizing the activity at one electrode common to a pair of channels. Thus LT (left temporal) is equal to all the activity at T_3, minus $\frac{1}{2}$ the activity at F_{p1} and O_1, etc. Negative events at T_3 produce upward deflections in the LT write-out.

Autospectral analysis of the secondary derivations was carried out on a TD 100 computer, averaging the spectra of three 10-sec epochs of each channel in each condition. Thus, for each derivation of each subject, power spectra were obtained for two conditions, 30 sec eyes open and 30 sec eyes closed.

Spectra were then integrated with respect to frequency, and these numbers were printed out by the computer after conversion to decimal form. Total power was next divided into four frequency bands by subtraction of the integral values at the lowest frequency of each band from the higher frequency limit. The four frequency bands were as follows: delta, 0.5–4 Hz; theta, 4–8 Hz; alpha, 8–14 Hz; beta, 14 Hz and higher.

To display results, the numerical value of power in each frequency band of each spectrum was plotted manually as a bar of proportional number of figures of the appropriate anatomical position on a circle representing the head (see Figs. 2–4). By using different figures for the eyes-open and eyes-

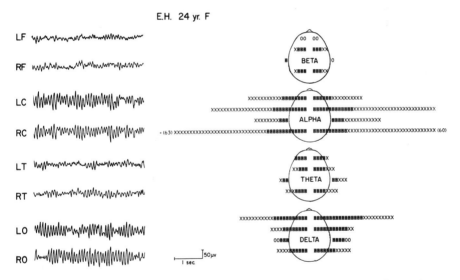

FIG. 2. EEG and display of spectral results from a normal subject. The EEG sample was obtained from secondary derivations as illustrated in Fig. 1.

Each head diagram on the right represents the total spectral power in the frequency band indicated during three 10-sec epochs with eyes open and three 10-sec epochs with eyes closed. The numbers of figures at each anatomical site are proportional to the spectral power recorded from that site in the specified frequency band. Results during eyes open (O's) are superimposed upon those with eyes closed (X's).

Guidelines for interpretation are given in the text. At a glance, one can see that alpha activity is maximum posteriorly and that there is more of it with the eyes closed (X's) than open (O's). The large amount of delta activity in the front of the head is believed to be eye-movement artifact.

B.J. 33 yr. F.

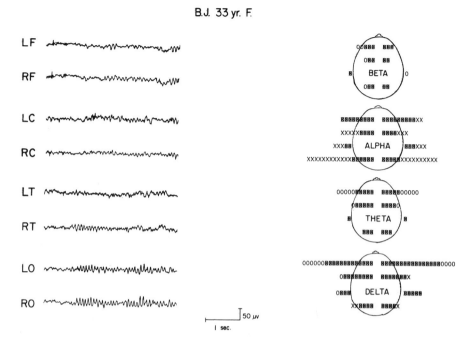

FIG. 3. EEG and analytical display from another normal subject. This is a much lower voltage EEG than the one illustrated in Fig. 2. Again, slow activity (delta and theta) in the front of the head is probably eye-movement artifact.

closed conditions (O and X, respectively), spectral results for these two conditions were superimposed on the display. Complete display of all values for one subject were thus represented on one page containing four spectro-anatomical graphs, one for each frequency band.

RESULTS

Displays of the analysis results are illustrated in Figs. 2–4, along with a 4-sec sample of the raw EEG data (secondary derivations).

Guidelines for interpretation of these displays are quite similar to those used for viewing conventional EEGs, except that the interpreter is not required to determine frequency, which is given by the analysis and printed out, and the time dimension is eliminated by averaging relatively long epochs and presenting this average as one static display representing 60 sec of data (30 sec eyes open and 30 sec eyes closed).

The interpretation should proceed as follows. First, examine the alpha

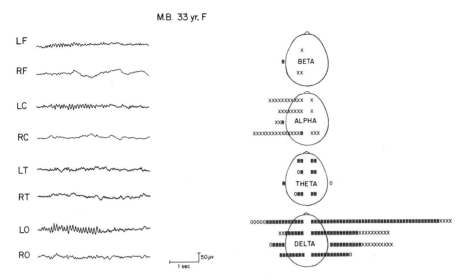

FIG. 4. EEG and analytical display from a patient with proven arteriovenous malformation involving the right frontal lobe. Note the marked asymmetry of beta and alpha activity and the presence of excessive delta activity over the right side, maximum in the right frontal area.

rhythm. It should be the major frequency in terms of total power; maximum posteriorly; reactive to eyes opening (many more X's than O's) fairly symmetrical in left versus right homologous positions (not more than twice the amount on one side as compared to the other). Note that this guideline is fulfilled in Figs. 2 and 3 (normals), but not in Fig. 4 (abnormal). In Fig. 4, the alpha activity is almost completely absent over the right hemisphere.

Next look at the beta activity. This is a normal frequency if it has less power than the alpha band; it should also be fairly symmetrical on the two sides of the head; it does not change much from the eyes-open to eyes-closed state. Note that in Fig. 4 beta activity is present on the left but absent on the right, another abnormal feature of this record.

Next observe the theta plot. A small amount of theta is usually present in all normal records; it should be less than the alpha in abundance and should be symmetrical on the two sides. If the amount of theta activity exceeds the alpha by inspection, one should suspect abnormal slowing of the EEG, which implies diffuse disturbance of cerebral function. In Fig. 3 (normal) there is an unusual amount of theta activity in frontal leads when eyes are opened. Some of this may be eye-movement artifact, but even if real, it is not considered to be significant because it does not exceed the alpha in this location.

Lastly, the delta band is examined. It is also abnormal if it exceeds the amount of alpha activity. These plots show a surprisingly large amount of delta activity in the normal subjects, particularly in frontal leads. There are several possible explanations: spectral technique, long-time constant employed and eye-movement artifact. It is clear, however, that Fig. 4 shows excessive delta activity over the entire right hemisphere, maximum in the right frontal area with eyes opened and closed; this finding indicates a localized disturbance or a lesion involving the right frontal area. The combination of depression of alpha activity and abnormal slow (delta) focus suggests acute or destructive lesion.

Obviously, guidelines for interpretation of such plots can be greatly sharpened, qualified and expanded as experience with the technique is gained by correlating the plots with results of conventional EEG and with other clinical/pathological findings.

DISCUSSION

This EEG analysis and display system involved many time-consuming elements, such as tape recording, channel-by-channel analysis off-line, print out and subtraction of numbers, and manual plotting of data, but such a system could be automated easily with existing techniques and hardware. The resulting transformation of conventional multi-page, multi-channel EEG data, which take years to learn to interpret, offers the following advantages: (1) a simplified, anatomically arranged display of clinical EEG data on a single page which can be interpreted easily by a clinician without extensive specialty training; (2) test results that are more objective and quantifiable, increasing reproducibility and improving diagnostic accuracy; (3) a system which is amenable to time- and distance-saving techniques, using electrode helmets (Frost, 1970), telephone transmission, and central computer facilities, which results in a high volume of tests available to large population areas at a low cost per test.

If automated in its present form, this system would be most useful as a screening test for adults and adolescents who are referred for many of the common reasons for obtaining an EEG, such as headaches, dizzy spells, psychiatric problems, and minor head injuries. The tests could reasonably be expected to reveal the presence of any gross lesion or disturbance and to free the electroencephalographer from the task of paging through immense numbers of probably normal EEGs looking for evidence of one or two unsuspected cerebral lesions among a thousand or so referrals. Seriously ill or comatose patients and those with definite neurological problems such as epilepsy, however, should receive conventional EEGs because waveform information, certain brief transients and dynamic changes in EEG during the test are ignored by the screening technique. Some of these aspects could eventually be built into the screening procedure, and suitable automatic techniques are already being tested (Saltzberg, Heath and Edwards, 1967; Buckley, Saltzberg, and Heath, 1968; Carrie, 1971.)

Since this feasibility study was begun over a year ago, a similar approach has been reported by Bickford (1971) and Bickford, Fleming, Billinger, Stewart and Aung (1971). The goal of Bickford's project is the same—production of a simplified one-page display of EEG analyzed by spectral technique. Bickford's system is, however, more comprehensive in that several minutes of EEG data are represented with serial three-dimensional plots of smoothed raw spectra. In spite of the advantage of retaining the dynamic aspects of EEG (which I do not feel are essential for screening tests), Dr. Bickford's displays seem to burden the interpreter with the difficulties of reading spectrograms. For screening purposes, division of the spectra into four cardinal frequency bands as illustrated here obviates the necessity of visual assessment of complex graphs and simulates part of the role of the electroencephalographer. Compression of time by averaging spectra further simplifies and quantifies the interpretation. The display presented in this system has the advantage of representing two different physiological states simultaneously—eyes open and eyes closed. Such attention to reactivity or lack of it is very helpful clinically. Even the procedure of recording these two states insures constant vigilance on the part of the patient and decreases errors of interpretation due to drowsiness. Of course, this could be easily incorporated in Dr. Bickford's procedure. As an ideal system, one could display the entire spectrum in Bickford's format along with a time summary in four bands as illustrated here, gaining the most from both types of display.

The montage employed in this system deserves further mention and discussion, since, to our knowledge, this technique has not been previously reported. Ideally, a monopolar or referential montage is preferable because of the straightforward information it provides about voltage distribution, but no universally acceptable reference has yet been devised which can be used for all areas of the head simultaneously without objectionable artifact, particularly EKG artifact. Bipolar or differential montages are "clean," but entail ambiguity of voltage distribution and necessitate logic for detection of voltage gradients. A bipolar montage with wide inter-electrode distance was selected for this study as a compromise to retain fair estimation of voltage gradients. A bipolar montage with wide inter-electrode distance was selected for this study as a compromise to retain fair estimation of voltage distribution and elimination of artifact with a minimum number of electrodes for eight different scalp areas. Secondary derivations from the original montage improve the ability to separate areas of the scalp and thereby simulate "monopolar" records.

The choice of spectral analysis was simply for convenience; the computer used (TD 100) is already programmed for this technique. The same results could as easily be obtained by period analysis with subsequent sorting into broad period bins corresponding to the appropriate frequencies plotted here. Frequency analysis could also be carried out with broad-band filters.

SUMMARY

This chapter describes and gives initial test results of a simple system for analyzing multi-channel clinical EEG data and displaying the results on one page in an anatomical format which can be easily comprehended by physicians having little formal training in electroencephalography.

Eight-channel clinical EEGs were submitted to spectral analysis (autospectra of each channel in eyes-open and eyes-closed conditions), and the spectral results were then divided into four cardinal frequency bands: beta, alpha, theta, and delta. The display consists of four figures of the head (one for each frequency band) upon which are plotted bar graphs of the power of activity at appropriate anatomical locations.

This technique is illustrated with EEGs from two normal subjects and one abnormal patient. Elementary guidelines for interpreting the displays are given and possibilities for further development are discussed.

It is concluded that this technique could be easily automated to provide an inexpensive mass screening test for many routine EEG problems, but it is not intended to replace conventional EEG in complex neurological conditions.

ACKNOWLEDGMENTS

The authors gratefully acknowledge the technical assistance of Mrs. Norrie Saltzberg.

This work was partially supported by GRS Grant No. 66582, NIH Grant No. NS 04705, and by NIH Contract No. PH 43–68–1414.

REFERENCES

Bickford, R. G. (1971): As quoted in the condensed EEG opens a new era. *Medical World News*, June 11: 15–16.

Bickford, R. G., Fleming, N., Billinger, T., Stewart, L., and Aung, M. (1972): Use of compressed spectral arrays (CSA's) in clinical EEG. *Electroencephalography and Clinical Neurophysiology*, 33:245.

Buckley, J. K., Saltzberg, B., and Heath, R. G. (1968): Decision criteria and detection circuitry for multiple channel EEG correlation. IEEE Region III Convention Record, New Orleans, 26.3.1–26.3.4.

Carrie, J. R. G. (1972): An automatic detection and quantification system for spike-and-wave. *Electroencephalography and Clinical Neurophysiology*, 33:254.

Frost, J. D., Jr. (1971): EEG acquisition and processing in extra-laboratory environments. *Electroencephalography and Clinical Neurophysiology*, 31:303.

Saltzberg, B., Heath, R. G., and Edwards, R. J. (1967): EEG spike detection in schizophrenia research. *Digest of the 7th International Conference on Medical and Biological Engineering*, Stockholm, p. 266.

Automation of Clinical Electroencephalography.
Edited by P. Kellaway and I. Petersén.
Raven Press, New York © 1973.

Application of Compressed Spectral Array in Clinical EEG

Reginald G. Bickford, John Brimm, Lee Berger and Maung Aung

Department of Neurosciences, University of California, San Diego, School of Medicine, La Jolla, California 92037

Communication of information between electroencephalographer and clinician via the conventional EEG report often proves to be an unsatisfactory procedure. Although an EEG record classification such as the Mayo System (Bickford and Klass, 1963), improves communication, the neurologist is still left poorly informed, as compared, for instance, to the cardiologist's comprehension of his patients heart action after viewing the EKG tracing. It is felt that this problem can now be largely overcome by the medium of a pictorial EEG, the compressed spectral array (CSA; Bickford, Fleming and Billinger, 1971), which can be viewed at the bedside by the neurologist in the form of a single-page report.

METHOD

The power spectral analysis method used to process the EEG data is shown in Fig. 1. The EEG recorded by conventional electrodes and montage techniques from 8 to 16 channels is digitized (128 samples per second) by a PDP-12 computer (8K memory). Power spectra (Bickford, 1961; Walter and Brazier, 1969) are generated using a Fast Fourier program, and the components (usually 0.25 Hz to 16 Hz with 0.25 Hz resolution) are subjected to smoothing and displayed with override suppression on a digital plotter. Each line of spectra is generated from 4 sec of primary EEG data.

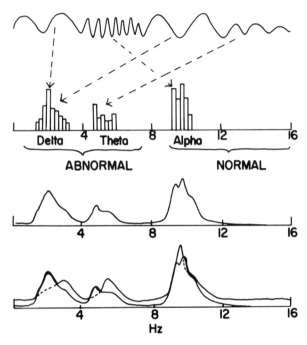

FIG. 1. Row 1 shows the original EEG tracing with mixed pathologic and normal frequencies. These are resorted during power spectral analysis, which tends to separate abnormal from normal frequencies since the former tend to be at the lower end of the spectrum in the waking state. The power spectrum is now smoothed (row 3) in preparation for the plotting process shown in Row 4. Here spectra from successive 4-sec periods of primary data are compressed sequentially down upon each other using the technique of "hidden-line suppression." This technique ensures that no subsequent line spectrum crosses a previously plotted spectrum and thereby provides the display with three dimensions for easy comprehensibility. In the CSA type of display, time rises vertically in 4-sec spectral increments.

Since this sampling period can be varied within wide limits (e.g., 8, 16, 32 sec), any desired degree of data compression can be achieved at the cost of discrimination.

RESULTS

An example of a alpha display from four different normal subjects is shown in Fig. 2. The ability of the display to follow serial frequency changes is evident when a sleep record is processed by this technique, as shown in Fig. 3. Note the disappearance of the alpha rhythm during drowsiness and the reappearance of an alpha-like frequency in the later part of sleep when

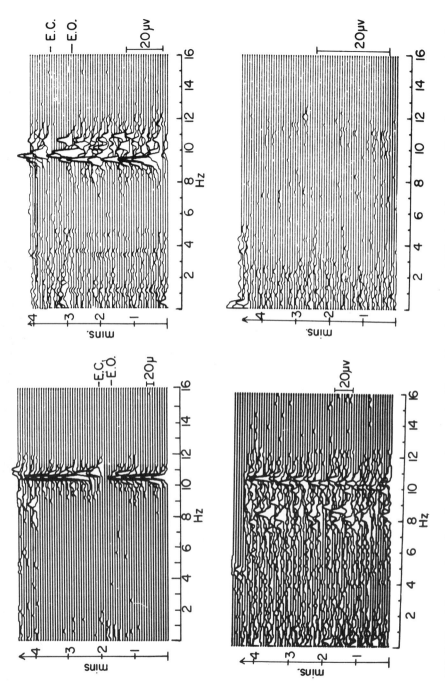

FIG. 2. The alpha spectrum from four separate normal subjects. Note the great variability in alpha spectra. The cleanest spectrum is shown on the *upper left*. In the *upper right* there is a wider spectrum; the *lower left* shows a bimodal alpha spectrum; and the *lower right* shows little activity in the alpha band (C_z–O_z).

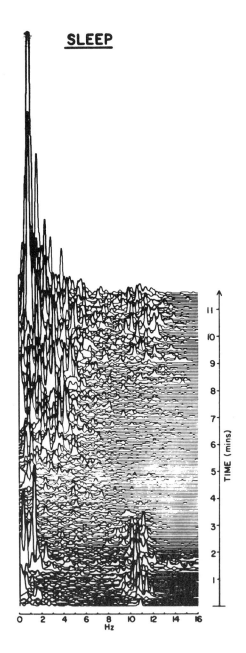

FIG. 3. A compressed spectrum from a single-channel EEG (C_z–O_z) in normal subject going to sleep. In the lower part of the spectrum the subject is awake and shows alpha rhythm and some eye blink artifact. At approximately 4 min, he becomes drowsy, with disappearance of the alpha rhythm, followed by increasing slow activity from 6 min onward as he passes into slow wave sleep. Note the reappearance of some alpha-like activity at 10 min.

predominant slow activity is present. The dynamic qualities of the display become even more evident when the response to photic stimulation is studied. An example is shown in Fig. 4, in which the light flash rate is progressively increased so that it sweeps smoothly across the frequencies quantitated in the spectrum (1–16 Hz). Note the compact summary of the persons' photic response obtained with this technique.

When single-channel spectra are arrayed in the relative positions from which they were sampled on the head, a highly informative display of EEG frequency related to space and time is obtained (see Fig. 5). In this adult record the symmetry of the alpha rhythm can be estimated, and an observer would be confident that the record was both reliable and normal. The method provides equally succinct display of the pathologic EEG. A section of the

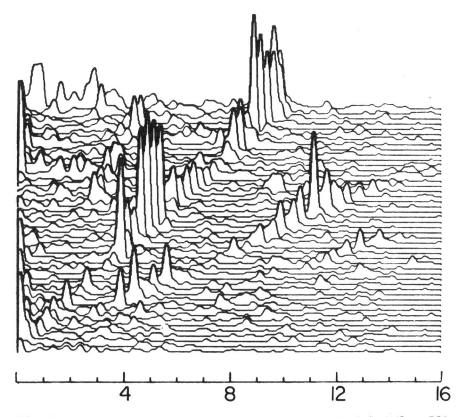

FIG. 4. Photic sweep. A C_z–O_z EEG recording of the response to photic flash (Grass PS2 at $I = 8$) in a normal subject. Response at the flash frequency is shown by the diagonal response peaks of 4 and 10 Hz. A divergent series of peaks can also be seen below the main peaks which represent the second harmonic response.

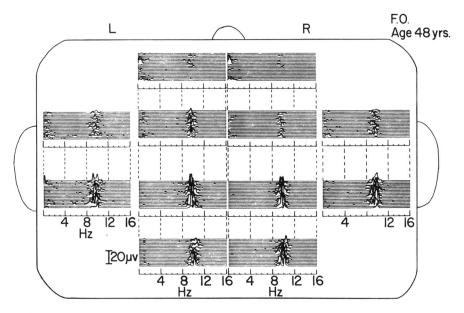

FIG. 5. Shows the compressed spectral array from a 12-channel EEG of a normal subject (bipolar montage). Note the symmetric alpha rhythm in the lower six arrays and an asymmetry of the mu-like rhythm in the motor regions. There is no appreciable slow activity present.

primary EEG tracing from which the CSA was made is shown in Fig. 6. Thus, a focal delta abnormality occurring in an infant is shown in Fig. 7. Note how easily the CSA can be read and the location of the abnormality recognized. The child had a birth defect with a cyst in the left temporal area.

An example of a generalized delta abnormality is shown in Fig. 8; a sample of the primary EEG data from which the CSA was made appears in Fig. 9. Note the contrast of this adult record with that of the normal adult shown in Fig. 5. The normal alpha process is obliterated, and the presence of high-voltage slow activity in all head regions is clearly evident in the 16-channel CSA.

DISCUSSION

The clinical CSAs that have just been discussed illustrate well the compression of clinical EEG data which is possible by this technique. It is also evident that the CSA lends itself to relatively easy comprehension by those who have had no more than perhaps a superficial exposure to the main

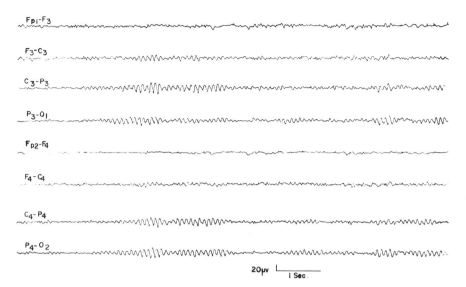

FIG. 6. An excerpt from the primary EEG recording on the subject whose CSA is shown in Fig. 5 (age 48 years).

abnormalities that are encountered in clinical practice. Its successful application, however, requires great care in recording technique to avoid artifact, particularly that encountered with eye movement. A limitation of the system, described above, is its inability to detect spike or sharp wave discharges except when they are accompanied by a slow wave. To meet this problem, a special program has been designed which will allow continuous monitoring and recognition of spike discharges in all 16 channels recorded. When a recognition is made, an asterisk is placed at the end of the appropriate spectral line on the CSA. Further developments will be necessary before the system can be used on complex EEG records. At present, it will process effectively 50% of records coming from an average EEG laboratory. With anticipated changes in recording and processing techniques, a continuing improvement in operation on the more complex records is expected.

The question of the economic feasibility of a system for clinical EEG recording using presently available computer technology can be answered in the affirmative. Using a mini-computer and a moderate amount of core storage (16K) and output via a storage tube and hard copy device (such as the Tektronix 1410 System), a system can be built for a rental of approximately $4.00 for each EEG run on the CSA system, (assuming a 5-day re-

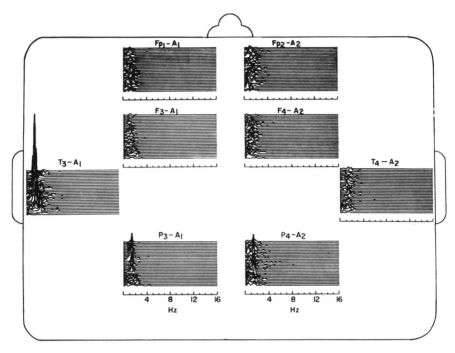

FIG. 7. CSA on an infant with a congenital malformation (cyst formation) in the left temporal area. Note the clearly defined slow-wave delta discharge appearing from the left temporal region. No adult type of alpha peak is seen since the patient was an infant. Bipolar montage.

cording week and eight EEG records processed per day). Such a system has the added advantage of providing the electroencephalographer with a powerful, general purpose computer which can be used effectively in EEG research when it is not occupied by clinical processing.

SUMMARY

A new system for the pictorial display of frequency information contained in the clinical EEG is described. The method can be used to compress EEG information on a 30 to 40 min clinical recording onto a single page. In addition to frequency information, there is continuous monitoring of 16 channels for identification of spike transients, the recognition of which is recorded on the arrayed spectra. The CSA is easily interpreted and economically feasible with the use of present mini-computer and oscilloscope copy technology.

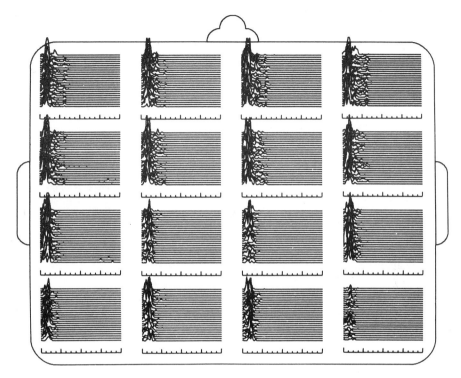

FIG. 8. A 16-channel CSA in a patient, age 24 years, showing generalized delta activity resulting from a cardiorespiratory arrest. Bipolar montage.

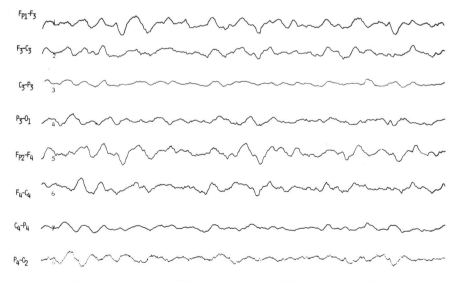

FIG. 9. Excerpt from EEG of patient whose CSA is shown in Fig. 8.

ACKNOWLEDGMENT

This work was supported by U.S. Public Health Service Grants NS–08961–04 and NS–08962–04.

REFERENCES

Bickford, R. G. (1961): Scope and limitations of frequency analysis. *Electroencephalography and Clinical Neurophysiology*, 20:9–13.

Bickford, R. G., Fleming, N. I., and Billinger, T. W. (1971): Compression of EEG data by isometric power spectral plots. *Electroencephalography and Clinical Neurophysiology*, 31:631–636.

Bickford, R. G., and Klass, D. W. (1963): Electroencephalography. In: *Clinical Examinations in Neurology*, Vol. 6, edited by members of the Sections of Neurology and Physiology, Mayo Clinic and Mayo Foundation for Medical Education and Research, Graduate School, University of Minnesota. W. B. Saunders Co., Philadelphia, pp. 297–310.

Walter, D. O., and Brazier, M. A. B. (1969): Advances in EEG analysis. *Electroencephalography and Clinical Neurophysiology, Supplement No. 27*. Elsevier Publishing Co., Amsterdam.

Automation of Clinical Electroencephalography.
Edited by P. Kellaway and I. Petersén.
Raven Press, New York © 1973.

Wavelength-Amplitude Profile Analysis in Clinical EEG

J. R. G. Carrie and J. D. Frost, Jr.

Neurophysiology Department, Methodist Hospital and Baylor College of Medicine, Houston, Texas 77025

The results of EEG analysis techniques such as power spectral and coherence analysis cannot be interpreted clearly and easily by most clinical electroencephalographers within the conceptual framework that they use in describing what they see in EEG recordings. We have developed a system for clinical EEG quantification which employs wavelength-amplitude analysis because, in our view, this type of analysis simulates some aspects of the process of human visual EEG interpretation. A consideration of the way in which a human electroencephalographer assesses the frequency and amplitude characteristics of an EEG tracing suggests that he estimates the number of complete waves in a standard interval of time and the peak-to-peak amplitude of those waves. A more detailed discussion of this approach has been published elsewhere (Carrie and Frost, 1971).

In developing our system for clinical EEG quantification, the following objectives were kept in view: (1) the hardware should be standardized and readily available; (2) the operating procedures should be simple, so that a technician could learn to use the system with a short period of instruction and supervision; and (3) the output of results should be rapid enough to allow on-line modification of the clinical investigation or experimental procedure.

METHOD

Frost (1969) has described a prototype system, and Carrie and Frost (1971) have given a detailed description of a later and more versatile system.

65

As outlined below, the current version includes further refinements in methodology, and a number of technical improvements have been incorporated.

Data Acquisition

Two channels of EEG are analyzed simultaneously, either directly on-line or off-line from magnetic tape. The amplified signals operate a conventional pen-recorder and are also sent through lines to the computer room. After analog bandpass filtering, the signals enter the input of a LINC-8 computer. By detecting positive-going baseline crossings, the digital program sorts consecutive EEG waves in a given frequency band into 60 different wavelength categories and counts the waves in each category. It also computes the summated peak-to-peak amplitude of the waves in each wavelength category. The programs can be adjusted to sample for a given period of time or for a specified number of waves and to cover different wavelength (frequency) ranges.

Statistical Analysis and Graphic Display

Information from each analysis run is stored on a single LINC tape-storage block. Before the analysis period, subject identification, such as name, EEG number and age, is typed in through the keyboard and is stored on the same block used for the EEG waveform analysis information. Data retrieval and analysis programs are used subsequently to locate information stored on particular blocks or under specified names. When the subject identification information is retrieved, the investigator has the option of selecting a statistical or graphic printout or of going straight to a clinical EEG descriptive printout. (Examples of the outputs from the analysis and display programs are given under Results.)

The graphic plots can be typed out on a Teletype Typewriter interfaced with a LINC-8 or a PDP-12 or on an Info-Max 57 Printer/Plotter interfaced with the PDP-12. Output is more rapid on the PDP-12/Info-Max system. The printout of a complete set of the histograms derived from the analysis of one channel during one analysis run takes 52 sec. The computation and printout of the relevant statistical variables take 45 sec.

Preliminary Automatic EEG Report

A clinical EEG report usually consists of a descriptive report in which the electroencephalographer describes the characteristics of the EEG waveform and an interpretive section in which he assesses the clinical significance of the findings. At the present time a preliminary automatic descriptive report and a limited interpretive report are provided by this system. Following computation of the quantitative characteristics of the EEG signal, information about the average wave amplitude on both sides, the handedness of the subject, the modal frequency on both sides, and about the number of waves at the modal wavelength on each side is used in automatically selecting and printing out an appropriate verbal report relating to the amplitude, symmetry and "degree of regulation" of the alpha rhythm. Currently, the criteria of abnormality in amplitude, and of symmetry in amplitude and frequency, have been determined somewhat arbitrarily by means of discussions with clinical electroencephalographers. For example, an EEG is rated as showing an abnormally low voltage if the average wave amplitude is less than 8.5 μV. A difference in frequency of 1.5 Hz between the two sides is considered abnormal. In view of the comments of Cobb (1963) regarding the significance of alpha asymmetry, a relative amplitude reduction of 50% over the dominant hemisphere is rated abnormal, whereas a reduction of 10% over the non-dominant hemisphere is classified abnormal. Categories relating to the "degree of regulation" of the alpha activity are based on an electro-clinical correlative study described below.

RESULTS

Wavelength-Amplitude Analysis of Typical EEG

Histograms. The graphic display programs provide plots of the EEG information acquired during the relevant analysis period. These plots show the number of waves in each wavelength category, the summated peak-to-peak amplitudes of all the waves in each category, and the mean wave amplitude in each category. Examples of these graphic plots are shown by Carrie and Frost (1971, Fig. 4).

Statistics. Figure 1 shows a printout of 17 variables that define the characteristics of the EEG waveform from one channel during one analysis run.

Correlation Between Automatic System and Human Electroencephalographer

The output from the prototype system consisted of a histogram showing the number of waves in each wavelength category. This system was used to examine the degree of correlation between one automatic measurement of the alpha activity and relevant elements in verbal reports provided by a

```
ALPHA ANALYSIS/LEFT


SUMMATED PEAK/PEAK AMPLITUDES
DURING DATA ACQUISITION= 15287 MICROVOLTS


MEAN WAVE AMPLITUDE/WAVELENGTH
PROFILE ANALYSIS...

WAVELENGTH OF WAVES WITH
LARGEST MEAN AMPLITUDE= 0096 MILLISECS

LARGEST MEAN AMPLITUDE= 0020.2 MICROVOLTS

MEAN= 0102 MILLISECS

VARIANCE= 0786 MILLISECS

STANDARD DEVIATION= 0028 MILLISECS

MEDIAN= 0094 MILLISECS

INTER-QUARTILE RANGE= 0028 MILLISECS

WAVECOUNT/WAVELENGTH
PROFILE ANALYSIS...

WAVECOUNT AT MODAL WAVELENGTH= 0126 WAVES

MODAL WAVELENGTH= 0086 MILLISECS

MEAN= 0088 MILLISECS

VARIANCE= 0133 MILLISECS

STANDARD DEVIATION= 0012 MILLISECS

MEDIAN= 0084 MILLISECS

INTER-QUARTILE RANGE= 0008 MILLISECS

ANALYSIS TIME= 0090 SECS

AVERAGE WAVE AMPLITUDE= 0015.3 MICROVOLTS
```

FIG. 1. Printout of 17 variables that define the characteristics of the EEG signal in one channel during a single analysis run.

human observer on the basis of visual inspection of tracings of the same EEG signals.

Sixty-six EEGs were recorded with the use of standard clinical recording techniques and were analyzed by a clinical electroencephalographer and also by the automatic system.

Firstly, a correlation coefficient of +0.80 was found between the dominant frequency specified by the electroencephalographer by visual inspection of the EEG records and the modal alpha wavelength defined by the automatic system.

The second type of correlation involved the number of waves of modal wavelength in the samples taken from the series of EEGs. Since the number of waves of modal wavelength is one indicator of the "stability" or "degree of regulation" of the most prominent alpha component, it was predicted that there would be a correspondence between this measurement and the relevant elements in verbal reports based on visual assessment. An experienced electroencephalographer provided verbal reports on each EEG recording without knowledge of the type of analysis to which his assessments would be subjected. It was found that the verbal reports could be divided into four categories with regard to content describing the alpha-activity "stability." The average numbers of waves of modal wavelength in 1,000-wave samples in these four groups differed. A Mann-Whitney U-Test showed that these differences were highly significant when the groups categorized as showing "poorly sustained" or "uncountable" alpha rhythms on visual assessment were compared statistically with the group whose alpha frequency was stated without any comment on the alpha-waveform stability.

These results suggested that the automatic system was at least in some respects simulating the performance of a human electroencephalographer.

Preliminary Automatic EEG Report

Figure 2 shows the stored clinical information and the descriptive alpha printout relating to a normal EEG. Figure 3 shows the alpha report derived from the EEG of a hypertensive patient who had a somewhat poorly organized EEG showing small amplitude.

Clinical Pharmacology

In addition to developing this wavelength-amplitude analysis technique as a basis for automatic EEG interpretation, we have used this system in an investigation of the effects of flurazepam hydrochloride (Dalmane®) on the waking EEG (Frost *et al.*, 1973).

The EEG detected at the occipital and central electrodes referred to the ipsilateral ears was subjected to computer analysis. No consistent changes were seen in the alpha or theta activity. The most consistent changes were seen in beta activity detected at the central electrodes. The effect of the drug on three of the seventeen variables that are computed by the analysis pro-

```
BLOCK NUMBER: 120

THE FOLLOWING IS NEW LABEL INFORMATION:

NAME: HOPKINS HENRY

EEG NUMBER:70-4105

DATE OF EEG: MAY 13,1970

AGE: 061 YEARS

HANDEDNESS: RIGHT

RIGHT ANALYSIS TIME: 090 SECONDS

TIME OF EEG: 09 AM

THE NEXT BLOCK SHARES LABEL INFORMATION WITH THIS BLOCK.

LEFT ANALYSIS TIME: 090 SECONDS


BLOCK NO. 120


OPTION NO. 2
                         ALPHA REPORT


 THE FINDINGS IN THIS EEG ARE WITHIN THE RANGE OF NORMAL VARIABILITY.
```

FIG. 2. "Alpha report" on normal EEG.

```
BLOCK NO. 010


OPTION NO. 2
                         ALPHA REPORT


 THE AMPLITUDE OF THIS EEG IS ABNORMALLY LOW ON BOTH SIDES.
 RIGHT SIDE=4718 UNITS
 LEFT SIDE=4770 UNITS

THIS EEG IS SOMEWHAT POORLY REGULATED ON THE LEFT SIDE.

THIS EEG IS SOMEWHAT POORLY REGULATED ON THE RIGHT SIDE.
```

FIG. 3. "Alpha report" on abnormal EEG.

gram for each channel are shown in Fig. 4. These variables are the mean wavelength, the average wave amplitude, and the number of waves during the 30-sec analysis time. The analysis covers the wavelength or frequency range between 14 and 38 Hz. Twelve samples were taken on a baseline day

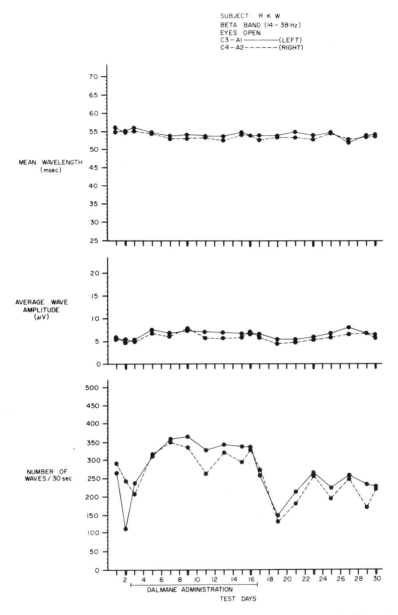

FIG. 4. Longitudinal plots showing increase in number of waves during fixed duration in 14–38 Hz range during administration of flurazepam hydrochloride, with no detectable change in mean wavelength or average wave amplitude. Heavy bars on horizontal axis show days on which 12 samples were taken for analysis, with results from single samples on intervening alternate days.

and then at weekly intervals during a 30-day study, with single-sample analysis on intervening alternate days. The drug was administered during the first 2 weeks following the baseline reading, and a placebo was given during the second 2 weeks. Figure 4 shows that there was no detectable change in the mean wavelength or average wave amplitude during the experiment. However, the number of waves in a standardized analysis interval increased while the drug was being administered.

Human visual interpreters who were concerned with reading the conventional EEG tracings detected a change in beta activity while the subjects were receiving the drug, and their interpretations showed a good correlation with those of the computer in defining the time course of this change. However, the electroencephalographers did not detect the change in the frequency of occurrence of the beta waves quite as sharply as the computer analysis system.

DISCUSSION

Several workers have used half-period measurements for EEG waveform analysis (Burch *et al.*, 1964; Tecce and Mirsky, 1967; Sulg, 1969). Full-period or wavelength analysis was used in the present system because it was considered that this method corresponded more closely to some aspects of the processing by a human electroencephalographer of the information contained in a tracing of an EEG signal. Legewie and Probst (1969) also used "wavelength-amplitude" or "period-amplitude" analysis, but there are several differences between the technique developed by Legewie and Probst and the system described here. The most important difference is the degree of resolution provided by the wavelength categorization process: whereas Legewie and Probst have only one wavelength category per Hertz unit, the present system uses substantially "narrower" categories, providing a greater degree of temporal resolution in the waveform analysis.

Throughout the development of this system, an attempt has been made to integrate it as practically as possible with the standard clinical recording situation. The initiation of an on-line real-time data acquisition program requires the technician merely to press a button on the recorder console and to note when the program terminates automatically by observing an indicator light. The process of data acquisition therefore interferes minimally with the usual recording procedure. It has been found that personnel with no previous experience in computer operation, such as EEG technicians and high school students, can learn to use both the data acquisition and the analysis program after only a short period of instruction and supervision. The rapid availability of the results of the analysis allows on-line flexibility in the organization of the research or clinical investigation.

At the present time, the criteria that are used by the automatic system in making judgments of normality and abnormality are preliminary and very incomplete. Additional information will be used by the program as it becomes available. In future developments, these programs will be used to obtain multivariate information about EEG characteristics from control subjects and several categories of patients. For diagnostic purposes, the probabilities of the multivariate results from a given individual being classified into each of the control and patient groups will then be computed using discriminant analysis techniques.

Although the automatic system and the human electroencephalographer have shown a high degree of correlation in describing several characteristics of EEG waveforms, at this stage it appears that it will be a long time before a computer system can match the human electroencephalographer in range and flexibility of performance. On the other hand, in our study of the effects of flurazepam hydrochloride on the EEG (Frost *et al., in press*), the change in the frequency of occurrence of waves in the beta frequency range without a change in wave amplitude was more clearly apparent in the output from the analysis system than on visual inspection of the EEG tracings. Thus it would seem that even at this early stage of development, the analysis system may be a useful supplement to the human specialist in certain particular and practical aspects of EEG waveform analysis.

SUMMARY

A method for quantitative wavelength-amplitude analysis of the EEG is described. The system has shown a high correlation with the human electroencephalographer in relation to some aspects of EEG evaluation and has defined some aspects of EEG waveform that were not immediately obvious to the human specialist. The operating procedures are easy to learn, and the prompt availability of quantitative results provides flexibility in application to clinical and research problems. The application of the technique to the development of a prototype automatic EEG analysis system and to clinical pharmacological research is described.

ACKNOWLEDGMENT

This investigation was supported in part by U.S. Public Health Service Grant HE 05435 from the National Heart Institute, and by Contract NAS 9–11120 from the National Aeronautics and Space Administration.

DISCUSSION

Walter and Saltzberg suggested that it might be of interest to study changes in the EEG variables measured by this technique using short analysis times such as 1 sec. It would be interesting, for example, to see whether the counts in the different wavelength categories increase in parallel or, on the other hand, in a serial manner, sometimes in one category, sometimes in another.

Kellaway commented that this technique gives a simple quantitative output that could be used in defining intrasubject EEG changes during aging that might be of diagnostic and prognostic significance regarding the development of certain diseases. It could also be of importance in defining changes in the physiological status of certain groups of patients such as those with abnormalities of cardiac function. For example, following the heart transplants performed at the Texas Medical Center, all of the transplant patients showed increases in their alpha frequencies. Similarly, Sulg has studied patients with cardiac pacemakers and has found that the correct functioning of the pacemaker has a considerable influence on the amplitude and frequency of the alpha rhythm.

REFERENCES

Burch, N. R., Nettleton, W. J., Jr., Sweeney, J., and Edwards, R. J., Jr. (1964): Period analysis of the electroencephalogram on a general-purpose digital computer. *Annals of the New York Academy of Sciences,* 115:827–843.

Carrie, J. R. G., and Frost, J. D., Jr. (1971): A small computer system for EEG wavelength-amplitude profile analysis. *Biomedical Computing,* 2:251–263.

Cobb, W. A. (1963): The normal adult E.E.G. In: *Electroencephalography: A Symposium on its Various Aspects,* edited by D. Hill and G. Parr. Macmillan, New York, p. 238.

Frost, J. D., Jr. (1969): Wavelength analysis of the EEG — The alpha profile. *Electroencephalography and Clinical Neurophysiology,* 27:702–703.

Frost, J. D., Jr., Carrie, J. R. G., Borda, R. P., and Kellaway, P. (1973): The effects of Dalmane (flurazepam hydrochloride) on human EEG characteristics. *Electroencephalography and Clinical Neurophysiology* 34:171–175.

Legewie, H., and Probst, W. (1969): On-line analysis of EEG with a small computer (period-amplitude analysis). *Electroencephalography and Clinical Neurophysiology,* 27:533–535.

Sulg, I. Z. (1969): The quantitated EEG as a measure of brain dysfunction. *Scandinavian Journal of Clinical and Laboratory Investigation,* Suppl. 109:23.

Tecce, J., and Mirsky, A. F. (1967): A system for off-line computer analysis of EEG amplitude and frequency. *Institute of Electrical and Electronics Engineers Transactions on Bio-Medical Engineering,* 14:202–203.

Automation of Clinical Electroencephalography.
Edited by P. Kellaway and I. Petersén.
Raven Press, New York © 1973.

Frequency Analysis of the EEG in Normal Children and Adolescents

Miloš Matoušek and Ingemar Petersén

Department of Clinical Neurophysiology, The Sahlgren Hospital, Göteborg, Sweden

Studies on the EEG of normal children from ages 1 to 16 years have recently been published by Petersén, Eeg-Olofsson, Hagne and Selldén (1965), Petersén, Eeg-Olofsson and Selldén (1968), and Petersén and Eeg-Olofsson (1971), and on the EEG of normal adolescents by Eeg-Olofsson (1971). The present study completes the results obtained in the preceding studies by visual analysis of records. Most EEGs were tape recorded, which enabled further data processing; this study deals with objective measurement of the background activity by means of broad-band frequency analysis. Some preliminary results had been published previously (Matoušek and Petersén, 1969; Petersén and Matoušek, 1971).

MATERIAL AND METHODS

Selection of Proper Subjects

The present material consists of the EEGs obtained from 401 children without mutual kinship (218 girls and 183 boys) and from 160 adolescents (85 females and 75 males). All details regarding the sampling of material have been described in the publications cited above.

The subjects have the following criteria of normality:

1. an uneventful prenatal, perinatal (gestational age not less than 37 weeks, birth weight above 2,500 g), and neonatal period

75

2. no disorders of consciousness
3. no head injury with cerebral symptoms
4. no history of central nervous system diseases
5. no obvious somatic diseases
6. no convulsions
7. no family history of convulsive disorders other than those secondary to acquired cerebral damage
8. no paroxysmal headache or abdominal pain
9. no enuresis or encopresis after the fourth birthday
10. no tics, stuttering, pavor nocturnus or excessive nailbiting
11. no obvious mental diseases
12. no conduct disorders
13. no deviation with regard to mental and physical development

For primary selection of subjects, a questionnaire was used. A detailed and standardized examination, with special regard to neurological status and psychic conditions according to a fixed schedule, was provided in selected subjects. Subjects belonging to the following categories were not excluded (in parenthesis number from the total $N = 401$ in children and $N = 160$ in adolescents):

1. exceptionally occurring syncopes connected with orthostatism, pain or fear ($N = 7$ in children and $N = 14$ in adolescents)
2. head injury without loss of consciousness or any other cerebral symptom ($N = 22$ and $N = 5$, respectively)
3. affective lability of small extent, no medical treatment necessary ($N = 32$ and $N = 14$, respectively)
4. nonhereditary neuropsychiatric disease in the family ($N = 60$ and $N = 13$, respectively)

EEG Recordings

The EEGs were recorded with either a Grass or a Kaiser electroencephalograph. In most cases eight channels were used for the EEG and two for recording eye movements. The 10–20 electrode system of the International Federation was used, with the customary longitudinal and transverse bipolar derivations. In all recordings one montage with a common reference lead (homolateral ear) was also used. The paper speed was 3 cm/sec, the time constant 0.3 sec, and the filter 70 Hz. The procedure was as follows.

Recording at rest usually occupied the initial 30 min of registration. Running notes have been made in the resting EEG regarding the occurrence of drowsiness or anxiety of the subjects.

Hyperventilation was then attempted in children aged 3 years or more. It was performed for 3 min. The children were encouraged to draw as deep breaths as possible, at a rate of approximately 20 per min.

The recording was stopped 2 min after hyperventilation. For frequency analysis, a 60-sec sample beginning after 90 sec of hyperventilation was chosen. Intensity of hyperventilation was evaluated using subjective criteria.

EEGs at rest, in most cases also during hyperventilation, photic stimulation and sleep were tape-recorded, using an 8- or 16-channel FM system. Visual evaluation was provided by repeated inspection of the EEG recordings.

Frequency Analysis

In each EEG recording, six epochs of 10-sec duration were analyzed. Epochs without artifacts were visually selected; rest recordings before starting any activation procedure were chosen. EEGs derived from seven pairs of leads (F7–T3, F8–T4, T3–T5, T4–T6, P3–O1, P4–O2 and C0–C4) were processed by means of a broad-band analog frequency analyzer. Six frequency bands correspond to the following frequencies: delta (1.5–3.5 Hz), theta (3.5–7.5 Hz), alpha 1 (7.5–9.5 Hz), alpha 2 (9.5–12.5 Hz),[1] beta 1 (12.5–17.5 Hz) and beta 2 (17, 5–25 Hz). The frequency response curves of the filters were checked before starting the analysis; they were flat with sharp cut-off at the above limiting frequencies. The broad-band LC filters were stable, and no tuning was necessary (for a detailed description, see Kaiser, Petersén, Selldén and Kagawa, 1964). The read-out circuits (integrators) were calibrated separately for each recording by means of a standard signal of constant voltage, which was tape-recorded together with the EEG signal. The frequency of the calibration signal was carefully checked with regard to the frequency response of each filter. The analyzed EEG signal was compared continuously with the original paper recording, to avoid technical artifacts.

Further Data Processing

The output values of frequency analysis were typewritten automatically and then punched on IBM cards together with clinical data and were processed by a digital computer (SAAB D-21). In this way, averages and standard deviations for individual age groups and a correlation matrix with labeled significance limits for the whole material were computed, for each

---

[1] When the term "alpha" is used without any index, a summated output value for alpha 1 and alpha 2 is understood.

EEG derivation. The EEG parameters are listed in Table 2 (below). Besides these parameters, coefficients of variation (standard deviation/mean) in each frequency band were calculated to estimate the variability in a 60-sec period (*i.e.,* from six epochs of 10-sec duration each). According to our previous experiences, quotients constructed from various output data of frequency analysis were used. The theta/alpha quotient correlated better than untransformed quantity of theta activity with the visual evaluation of theta activity in respective recordings in previous studies (Matoušek, 1967). The agreement with the conventional description of EEGs was still better, if a constant value was added to the denominator (Matoušek, 1968). A quotient constructed in this way should be understood as a pure, empirically stated parameter, without any necessary physiological background. In this study were quotients with varying correction values between 0 and 10 determined, but only the most typical results with theta/(alpha + 8) quotient are presented below.

The amounts of theta and alpha activity are expressed in units corresponding to peak-to-peak voltages of the sine calibration signal at the center frequency of the respective frequency band (in microvolts).

The symmetry of all parameters used was estimated by means of another type of quotient. It compared the size of both values occurring in two symmetrical EEG derivations. The lower value was divided by the higher one, regardless of the side of the head.

Statistical Treatment

The statistical treatment consisted in determining means and standard deviations in individual 1-year groups as well as for the entire group of children aged 1 to 15 years, and separately for adolescents aged 16 to 21 years. This separation was necessary to improve the information on events occurring only in one of these age groups. Furthermore, a correlation matrix with labeling of significance levels was calculated. For comparison of correlation coefficients, Fisher's z-transformation was used. To follow the age-dependent changes of intra- and inter-individual variability, a non-parametric test (rank-correlation) was applied.

RESULTS

EEG Frequency Patterns in Various Age Groups

The age-dependent changes of mean amplitudes are shown in Figs. 1 and 2, separately for four EEG derivations. As shown, delta activity decreases

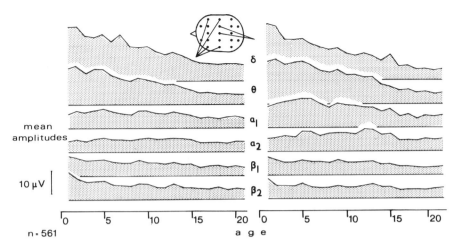

FIG. 1. Mean amplitudes in individual frequency bands related to age. Left: averaged output F7–T3 and F8–T4, right: derivation C4–C0.

nearly linearly with age. Theta and alpha 1 (7.5–9.5 Hz) activity both increase and culminate at approximately 4 and 8 years, respectively, then decrease again. Alpha 2 (9.5–12.5 Hz) activity increases continuously during childhood, and the amplitude level remains without prominent changes in adolescence. The amplitudes in beta frequency band decrease slightly with age. If the dominant activity (*i.e.*, the activity with relatively

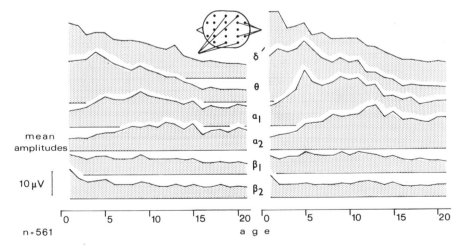

FIG. 2. The same as in Fig. 1, derivations T3–T5 and T4–T6 (left) and P3–O1 and P4–O2 (right).

TABLE 1. EEG activity in various frequency bands related to age (means and standard deviations of amplitudes in microvolts)

Age group	1–	2–	3–	4–	5–	6–	7–	8–	9–	10–	11–	12–	13–	14–	15–	16–	17–	18–	19–	20–	21–22
n =	19	18	18	22	26	18	26	41	25	31	24	29	29	49	26	26	32	21	29	25	27
F7–T3 & F8–T4																					
delta	23.6	23.6	19.2	18.9	19.9	16.6	15.0	14.7	14.2	14.6	12.6	11.2	12.0	10.2	8.7	7.8	7.5	7.1	7.5	7.4	6.8
	5.3	7.3	3.9	5.2	7.3	3.0	5.6	4.1	4.4	4.5	3.5	2.9	4.0	3.9	2.5	2.3	2.2	1.9	2.1	2.8	2.3
theta	15.4	16.9	13.8	15.0	15.1	12.5	11.1	10.2	11.2	10.8	9.9	8.5	8.8	7.4	6.2	4.9	5.2	4.4	4.7	4.3	4.2
	5.1	5.2	3.5	4.7	5.2	3.3	3.6	2.3	3.8	4.3	2.8	2.6	3.3	3.5	2.0	1.6	2.8	1.3	1.6	1.5	2.0
alpha 1	6.3	7.1	6.8	7.7	8.4	7.3	6.5	6.0	7.4	7.1	6.3	6.0	6.8	6.3	5.1	4.5	4.6	4.1	4.7	5.0	4.2
	1.9	2.0	2.5	2.3	3.1	2.4	1.8	1.7	3.6	3.8	2.6	2.6	3.6	5.0	2.4	2.4	2.8	2.0	3.2	3.0	2.2
alpha 2	4.8	5.1	4.8	5.3	6.0	5.4	5.2	4.9	5.3	5.4	5.1	5.3	5.5	5.4	5.4	3.8	3.9	4.1	4.0	4.6	4.3
	1.8	1.3	1.2	1.5	2.4	1.9	2.3	1.6	1.8	3.0	2.8	2.7	2.5	3.3	2.3	2.3	1.7	1.9	2.3	2.4	2.3
beta 1	8.4	7.4	6.5	6.7	6.9	5.9	5.5	5.3	6.3	5.5	5.2	4.9	5.5	4.8	4.6	3.9	4.0	4.5	3.7	4.1	3.4
	3.5	2.3	1.6	2.2	3.2	1.5	1.4	1.4	1.8	2.4	1.4	1.8	3.3	2.6	1.4	1.4	1.3	1.8	1.0	2.3	1.2
beta 2	11.7	8.6	7.5	7.7	7.9	6.2	5.9	5.6	6.4	6.4	5.2	5.0	6.4	4.9	4.6	4.7	4.4	5.6	4.2	4.9	4.5
	5.9	3.4	2.5	3.5	3.9	1.4	1.9	2.0	2.1	3.4	1.8	2.1	4.7	2.9	1.4	2.6	1.6	3.2	1.1	2.9	2.8
C0–C3																					
delta	24.4	24.0	17.7	17.1	17.7	15.9	14.1	13.5	13.6	11.9	10.7	11.1	10.5	8.2	6.7	6.0	6.1	4.7	4.8	4.2	4.8
	7.5	8.8	4.8	3.2	6.8	3.9	7.3	3.7	4.1	3.7	2.5	3.7	3.0	2.8	2.0	1.5	3.5	1.3	1.1	1.3	2.0
theta	18.2	19.4	16.8	17.5	18.0	16.6	14.0	13.6	14.8	12.2	12.4	11.1	11.3	8.5	7.7	5.8	6.0	4.8	5.1	4.4	4.9
	6.4	7.4	4.0	4.5	7.7	5.7	4.5	3.0	5.5	4.1	3.4	3.5	3.1	2.9	2.7	2.1	2.8	1.4	2.1	1.8	2.3
alpha 1	9.0	10.8	11.1	11.8	12.5	12.2	10.2	8.9	10.4	9.9	9.3	8.8	8.7	6.8	7.8	4.7	5.5	3.8	5.1	4.7	5.2
	3.6	6.4	5.0	4.6	5.1	6.5	4.0	3.1	5.2	6.4	4.0	5.3	4.7	4.1	4.5	2.5	4.2	1.6	4.0	2.8	3.9
alpha 2	5.7	6.0	6.7	6.5	8.8	8.4	6.9	7.7	7.8	7.9	7.3	9.2	9.2	6.7	9.0	4.6	4.6	4.6	5.3	5.0	5.3
	2.4	2.2	2.7	1.9	4.1	4.2	2.8	3.1	3.6	4.5	3.4	5.3	5.3	4.0	5.5	2.8	2.6	2.2	3.4	3.0	2.8
beta 1	7.9	6.5	5.8	5.8	6.2	5.8	5.6	5.4	6.2	5.1	5.3	5.8	5.5	4.4	4.7	3.7	3.7	3.5	3.3	3.4	3.7
	4.7	2.5	1.4	1.6	2.9	2.0	1.9	1.4	2.5	2.2	1.3	2.7	2.4	1.9	1.9	1.2	1.4	1.8	1.2	1.8	1.9
beta 2	8.8	5.8	5.5	5.2	6.1	4.9	4.8	4.7	5.4	4.9	4.7	5.3	6.1	4.4	4.9	3.8	3.8	3.8	3.8	4.3	4.5
	5.8	1.8	2.0	1.6	4.8	1.4	2.1	1.4	2.4	2.7	1.4	2.3	4.4	2.0	2.1	1.2	1.2	1.5	1.4	2.6	1.7
T3–T5 & T4–T6																					
delta	23.7	22.9	18.7	20.0	19.8	16.9	16.1	16.1	15.5	14.8	13.9	12.7	14.1	9.8	8.5	7.2	7.6	6.9	6.5	6.3	5.9
	6.8	5.3	4.7	6.5	6.7	4.6	6.0	7.2	5.7	5.6	4.7	4.4	11.7	3.8	3.0	2.4	3.4	2.0	2.2	2.0	2.3

theta	17.6	17.9	17.8	21.1	19.4	16.8	15.1	13.9	15.2	14.0	13.3	10.4	10.5	9.8	7.8	5.4	6.4	5.4	5.4	5.5	5.0
	7.7	7.7	5.0	8.1	7.0	7.5	5.6	6.3	6.1	6.1	6.5	4.2	3.7	5.0	3.6	2.2	4.6	1.8	2.7	2.8	2.7
alpha 1	6.7	7.4	8.2	10.5	13.4	11.1	11.1	12.5	15.0	13.2	12.4	11.6	10.1	9.3	9.6	7.2	8.9	7.9	7.6	9.0	8.0
	2.0	2.1	4.1	3.6	5.4	5.8	4.2	7.0	10.8	8.2	8.5	7.4	6.0	6.7	6.5	6.8	8.6	5.4	5.8	7.4	7.3
alpha 2	5.0	5.1	5.1	6.5	7.6	7.5	8.3	10.1	9.8	10.3	9.5	11.4	10.7	8.9	11.0	6.7	8.1	8.8	7.7	9.4	8.3
	1.5	1.5	1.4	2.6	3.0	3.4	4.7	5.8	4.2	8.0	5.5	7.4	5.1	4.5	5.5	4.8	5.0	5.3	5.9	5.0	4.8
beta 1	8.4	7.4	6.6	7.3	7.7	6.8	6.6	6.9	8.3	6.8	6.4	6.3	6.5	5.7	6.0	4.7	4.9	5.5	4.6	5.1	4.5
	2.8	2.7	2.0	2.7	3.5	2.5	1.6	3.1	2.3	2.8	2.0	2.7	2.9	2.2	1.8	1.7	1.9	3.2	1.3	2.4	1.6
beta 2	12.5	8.3	7.0	7.5	7.8	5.7	5.7	5.7	6.6	6.0	4.9	4.9	5.7	4.8	5.2	4.6	4.7	5.7	4.5	5.1	4.5
	6.7	3.4	2.4	3.7	4.3	1.5	1.7	2.7	2.2	2.7	1.5	2.0	3.6	2.1	1.5	2.0	1.8	3.2	1.5	1.8	1.6
P3–01 & P4–02																					
delta	28.3	20.1	28.3	21.7	23.4	18.0	19.2	16.7	16.8	16.8	16.4	13.9	13.4	11.1	9.3	7.5	7.4	7.0	6.3	6.9	6.1
	9.3	3.8	8.0	5.3	9.6	5.6	7.2	4.0	6.0	7.7	6.8	5.6	5.2	4.3	3.6	2.8	3.6	1.9	2.2	3.9	2.1
theta	19.0	21.1	22.5	22.4	25.6	21.7	17.7	16.5	18.0	16.7	17.0	12.6	12.6	10.1	9.6	6.6	7.0	6.5	6.2	6.3	5.8
	7.0	7.3	7.7	6.6	11.2	8.7	6.2	6.1	7.9	8.0	8.2	4.9	5.0	4.5	3.8	3.0	4.0	2.3	3.1	3.5	3.0
alpha 1	8.7	9.4	12.0	15.3	23.4	18.0	17.0	18.2	20.5	19.2	20.0	16.6	17.0	12.5	12.8	10.7	11.7	8.9	9.5	10.1	10.6
	3.3	3.3	6.1	5.3	12.2	6.7	7.0	7.3	10.3	9.6	11.7	9.2	9.0	8.3	7.4	10.0	9.2	5.8	6.5	7.6	8.5
alpha 2	5.7	6.0	6.8	7.9	11.0	11.1	11.6	14.5	14.0	14.4	15.1	17.8	18.8	13.5	16.6	12.4	12.8	11.8	11.4	13.1	13.1
	2.0	1.8	2.0	2.1	5.1	4.3	6.6	6.5	5.7	11.0	7.4	10.5	10.2	8.4	8.3	9.0	9.0	6.6	8.8	7.1	7.6
beta 1	7.3	6.0	7.1	7.3	9.0	8.0	7.5	7.7	8.9	7.7	8.5	8.4	8.0	6.6	7.2	5.8	5.3	6.1	5.1	5.4	4.8
	3.8	1.5	1.6	2.1	4.5	2.6	2.0	2.1	3.2	3.4	2.6	4.0	3.0	2.7	2.5	2.2	2.3	4.6	1.7	2.0	1.9
beta 2	9.1	5.9	5.7	5.5	6.2	5.2	5.3	5.5	5.9	5.6	6.2	7.0	6.8	5.2	6.5	4.9	4.5	4.9	4.6	5.5	5.1
	5.5	1.3	1.7	2.5	2.9	1.3	1.9	1.7	1.9	2.8	2.4	3.3	2.9	2.0	2.6	1.7	1.9	2.0	2.1	2.1	2.4

larger amplitude when compared with other frequency components) is studied separately, a subsequent substitution of the faster activity for the slower one may be demonstrated (Fig. 3).

The numerical information on mean amplitudes and their variability in individual 1-year age groups is summarized in Table 1. With one exception, the values are averaged for each pair of symmetrical EEG derivations.

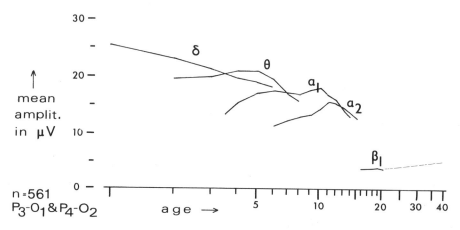

FIG. 3. Dominant activity in various age groups. The amount of beta activity approximated according to previous studies (Matoušek, Volavka, Roubíček and Roth, 1967).

The correlation of mean amplitudes and some derived parameters with age are summarized in Table 2. There are prominent differences between the groups of children and adolescents. The total amplitude (*i.e.*, the summated output values from all six frequency bands) decreases with age significantly during childhood, but the changes become insignificant in adolescence. Similar relationships may be observed in most individual frequency bands. Table 2 demonstrates also significant shifts of alpha activities, namely in favor of higher alpha frequencies in older subjects (alpha 1/alpha 2 ratio correlates negatively with age). Analogical changes appear in both beta frequency bands (beta 1/beta 2 ratio).

Topology

As a next step, the development of EEG activity in the course of maturation was studied separately in different EEG derivations and mutually compared. The parameter correlating in the highest degree with age (*i.e.*, an empirically stated quotient theta (alpha + 8); for details see Matoušek, 1968) is applied in Fig. 4 to demonstrate the topological differences. As shown, the

TABLE 2. Correlation between individual EEG parameters and age

Age	F7–T3, F8–T4 1–15	16–21	C0–C3 1–15	16–21	T3–T5, T4–T6 1–15	16–21	P3–O1, P4–O2 1–15	16–21
Quantities								
delta	−0.633*	−0.066	−0.692*	−0.264	−0.541	−0.187	−0.615	−0.145
theta	−0.611*	−0.130	−0.594*	−0.198	−0.512	−0.070	−0.504	−0.089
alpha 1	−0.135	0.024	−0.247	0.024	0.058	0.041	0.035	−0.022
alpha 2	0.034	0.108	0.129	0.107	0.309	0.116	0.398	0.023
beta 1	−0.361	−0.079	−0.262	0.005	−0.210	−0.011	0.001	−0.093
beta 2	−0.399	0.003	−0.179	0.174	−0.404	0.008	−0.056	0.105
Percentages								
delta	−0.421	−0.047	−0.581	−0.316	−0.601	−0.241*	−0.696*	−0.119
theta	−0.418	−0.205*	−0.364	−0.348*	−0.570	−0.182	−0.648	−0.131
alpha 1	0.354	0.055	0.069	0.059	0.342	0.038	0.246	−0.021
alpha 2	0.569	0.161	0.521	0.172	0.626*	0.175	0.660	0.097
beta 1	0.218	−0.086	0.338	0.067	0.234	−0.016	0.348	−0.078
beta 2	−0.044	0.015	0.306	0.333*	−0.178	0.045	0.226	0.183*
Quotients								
theta/alpha	−0.589	−0.178*	−0.439	−0.256	−0.670*	−0.182*	−0.703*	−0.066
theta/(alpha + 8)	−0.725*	−0.218*	−0.614*	−0.350*	−0.724*	−0.248*	−0.734*	−0.170*
beta 1/alpha	−0.280	−0.123	−0.098	−0.069	−0.324	−0.087	−0.244	−0.076
beta 2/alpha	−0.356	−0.040	−0.068	0.093	−0.484	−0.058	−0.363	0.060
delta/theta	−0.017	0.140	−0.272	−0.088	0.011	−0.119	−0.145	−0.060
alpha 1/alpha 2	−0.221	−0.099	−0.405	−0.138	−0.266	−0.089	−0.399	−0.054
beta 1/beta 2	0.229	−0.127	−0.097	−0.333*	0.362	−0.097	0.056	−0.212*
General amplitude	−0.524	−0.023	−0.475	−0.031	−0.308	0.011	−0.197	−0.034
$|\bar{X}|$	0.357	0.096	0.337	0.171	0.387	0.101	0.364	0.092

* Three highest correlation coefficients in each column.

changes proceed relatively fast in temporal and parieto-occipital derivations in the younger age groups. After reaching a point corresponding to the age of 8 years, approximately, the age-dependent decrease of the quotient slows down. Somewhat different relations may be seen in frontal and particularly in central derivations, where the decrease occurs more linearly over the entire age period 1 to 21 years. It follows that the age-dependent changes are relatively more pronounced in posterior derivations for children, and in anterior derivations for adolescents. For example, in subjects between 16 and 21 years of age, the quotient theta (alpha + 8) appears with age with correlation coefficient −0.350 in central and −0.170 in parieto-occipital derivations. The difference between coefficients is statistically significant ($P < 0.05$).

Similar significant differences have been obtained with most EEG parameters, particularly those dealing with theta activity. The amount of theta activity (expressed in percentages of the total EEG activity) correlate with age as follows:

	Derivation		
	Fronto-temporal		Parieto-occipital
1 to 15 years	−0.418	x	−0.648
	x		x
16 to 21 years	−0.205		−0.131

The x indicates a statistically significant difference between respective correlation coefficients (*P* < 0.01). Thus the decrease of theta activity with age is faster again in posterior EEG derivation, where younger age groups are concerned. Just the opposite trend, with faster decrease in anterior derivations, may be seen in older subjects.

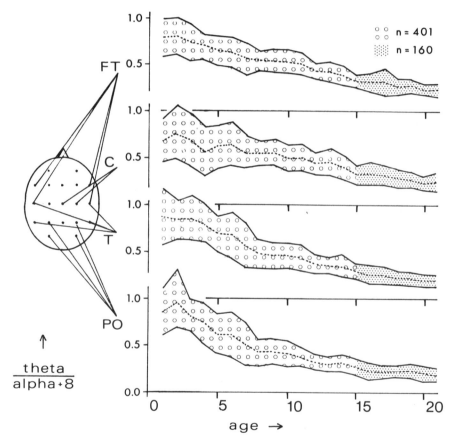

FIG. 4. Comparison of various EEG derivations. For demonstration we used an empirically constructed parameter which correlates in the highest degree with age.

The relationships among activities in anterior and posterior derivations were studied in another way, too. For each EEG parameter, a special ratio was calculated. It compared mutually the values corresponding to fronto-temporal and to parieto-occipital derivation. The lower value was divided by the higher one; thus, the size of the ratio was smaller when differences between respective recordings were more prominent. For theta activity (in percentages of the total EEG activity) and for all age groups, a mean ratio 0.79 with standard deviation 0.13 was obtained. It correlated significantly with age (correlation coefficient −0.279). The negative correlation meant that the differences between amplitudes of theta activity increased with age. Another EEG parameter is displayed graphically in Fig. 5 (lower part).

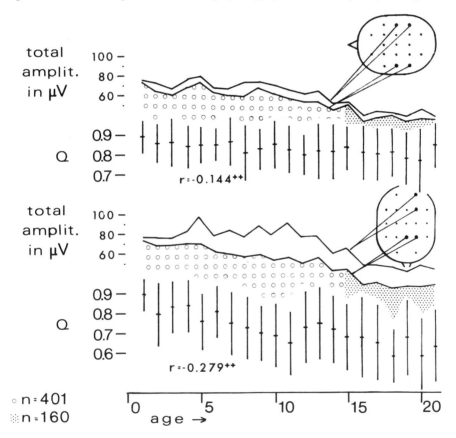

FIG. 5. Symmetry (upper part) and relationships between activities derived from anterior and posterior derivation (lower part). In each case, the summated amplitudes of all six frequency bands are shown in each of the paired derivations. Besides these, a ratio between the lower and higher value (mean ± standard deviation) is demonstrated as related to age.

The total amplitudes in two recordings are shown as two irregular curves. Below them are demonstrated means and standard deviations of the above-mentioned ratio, separately for each 1-year age group. The values of the ratio decrease significantly with age. Thus, the relative differences between amplitudes as they appear in respective EEG recordings become more prominent with age. Similar results may be obtained with other parameters, too. In summary, the differences between amplitudes in fronto-temporal and in parieto-occipital derivations are more pronounced in older subjects.

Symmetry of EEG Activities

As a rule, the amplitudes are larger on the sub-dominant hemisphere as has been stated by clinical examination (handedness judged from 3 years of age using criteria applied by Bingley, 1958). To eliminate the variability in connection with right- and left-handedness, a ratio dividing always the lower value by the higher one is used. In this way symmetrical EEG recordings are compared mutually for each subject and for each EEG parameter. The ratio approximates to 1.0 when the differences between two symmetrical derivations are minimal and becomes lower when some asymmetry appears. The results are similar in different frequency bands, and therefore a summated result may be obtained from the total EEG activity (Fig. 5, upper part). As shown, the asymmetry in temporal derivations increases significantly with age (*i.e.*, the ratio correlates negatively with age).

Some interesting results have been obtained by mutual comparing of various EEG parameters. The degree of symmetry is higher (*i.e.*, the ratio approximates to 1.0), and its variability is lower in relative parameters, where the amount of EEG activity is expressed as a percentage of some kind of quotient. Conversely, the untransformed output values of frequency analysis (corresponding to the amount or amplitude of respective EEG activity) have occurred very often with more prominent asymmetry, and the ratio has been more variable. The highest symmetry ratio may be obtained with theta activity expressed in percentages of the total EEG amplitude. The ratio averaged for all age groups reaches values between 0.91 and 0.92 with standard deviation 0.06–0.07 in all of three pairs of EEG derivations used.

The symmetry ratio is significantly higher in younger subjects. For instance, it correlates with age with correlation coefficient -0.116 in temporal derivations, in children between 1 and 15 years. In adolescents the age-dependent changes of symmetry become insignificant (analogical correlation coefficient -0.018), the ratio remaining still lower than in younger subjects.

Inter-Individual Variability

The inter-individual variability has been measured by coefficient of variation. The standard deviation is divided by the mean in each parameter, which is calculated for individual 1-year age groups. It informs on differences among various individuals within the same age group.

The variability is lowest in the theta frequency band, mean values of the coefficient being 0.37 in fronto-temporal, 0.34 in central, 0.44 in temporal and 0.42 in parieto-occipital derivations, respectively. The variability is highest in alpha frequency bands; corresponding values for alpha 1 activity are 0.52, 0.54, 0.59 and 0.57, respectively.

As demonstrated in Fig. 6 (upper curve), the inter-individual variability increases slightly but statistically significantly with age.

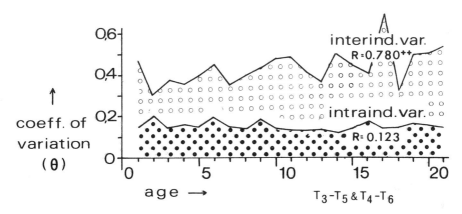

FIG. 6. Variability of theta activity related to age. Inter-individual variability (i.e., differences among individual within the same age groups) correlates significantly with age (upper curve), since the intra-individual variability (i.e., fluctuation of amplitudes during 60 sec of examination) does not correlate significantly. The significance is calculated with a nonparametric test for individual 1-yr age groups.

Intra-Individual Variability

The second type of variability regards fluctuation of EEG amplitudes as it appears during registration of brain activity. This is closely related to visually detectable modulation of EEG rhythms. The intra-individual variability has been computed from six successive epochs of 10-sec duration. A coefficient of variation has been stated in each subject, each EEG derivation and for each EEG parameter used. The obtained values are presented as averages, either for individual 1-year age groups, or for all examined subjects.

Such "60-sec variability" is lowest in beta 1 (*i.e.,* 12.5–17.5 Hz) frequency band. The coefficient of variation reaches values between 0.11 and 0.15 in each of EEG derivations used in this study. The variability is highest in alpha frequency bands, where values up to 0.28 may be obtained (age group 16 years, temporal derivations, alpha 2 frequency band). The respective values for delta and theta activity lie between these extremes, being slightly higher than those observed for beta activity (corresponding values 0.17 and 0.18, respectively).

The age-dependent changes of intra-individual variability are insignificant, if all age groups are taken into account (Fig. 6, lower curve). In fact, the intra-individual variability tends to decrease in children and increase in adolescents. Besides that, the dominating activity seems to occur with somewhat higher intra-individual variability than the other components. No details are mentioned here because the significance of these findings is doubtful.

Mutual Comparison of Various EEG Parameters

Most of the parameters used in this study correlate significantly with age, regardless of EEG derivation, frequency band and type of further transformation. The degree of correlation with age varies, however (Table 2). There is a clear preference for relative parameters, where the amounts of EEG activities are expressed in percentages or as quotients. The correlation is usually higher in those parameters dealing with delta or theta activity. As shown, the variations among different parameters are more clear in older age groups.

If the linearity or nonlinearity of observed relationships is comparable, the degree of correlation with age may be dependent on two factors: the respective change may occur more or less rapidly during ageing, or the correlation is reduced by increased variability of data. These various situations are demonstrated in Fig. 7. The untransformed quantity of theta activity (upper curve) is influenced considerably by the age factor, but the variability of data is relatively high. Therefore the correlation coefficient is lower than in remaining parameters. Just the opposite relationships may be noticed on the second curve, where the same values are expressed as percentages of the total EEG activity. Such a transformation reduces the variability significantly. According to our previous experiences, the quotients constructed from theta and alpha values are useful for statistical treatment of EEG data. A simple theta/alpha ratio (third curve) correlates

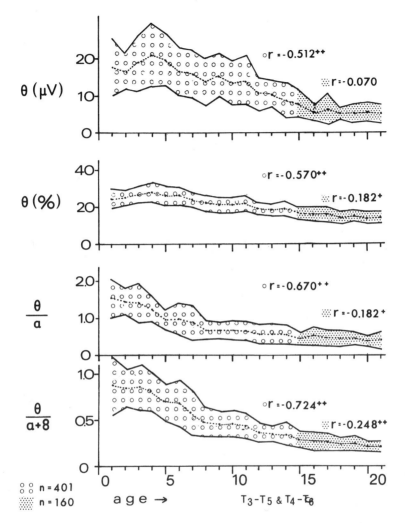

FIG. 7. Comparison of various EEG parameters: mean amplitude of theta activity, the same in percentages of the total EEG activity, theta/alpha quotient and similar quotient with an empirically stated correction. Note differences in variability and slopes of various curves as well as the size of correlation coefficients with age (separately for children and adolescents).

still better with age than previous parameters. An empirically stated value, "8", added to the denominator (Matoušek, 1968), improves further the degree of correlation (last curve). As shown in Table 2, this empirically constructed quotient occurs constantly with the highest correlation to age, regardless of EEG derivation and age category.

Frequency Analysis Compared with Visual Evaluation and Some
Non-EEG Items

To reduce the influence of age factor, the following correlations were
computed separately for children and for adolescents and presented mostly
only for the latter group.

Figure 8 (lower part) shows the correlation between amplitude of EEG
activity and an occurrence of visually judged abnormalities in the curve
(N = 16 from the total of 160 recordings). In EEGs with slight abnormalities
may be found a significantly increased amount of alpha 1 activity as well as
higher values of the total amplitude. The amount of beta 2 activity is somewhat lower in these recordings. Because the abnormal EEGs appear
randomly in various age groups, it is of some interest to compare the mentioned deviations with age-dependent changes of the frequency pattern (Fig.
8, upper part). The age factor influences significantly delta, theta and alpha

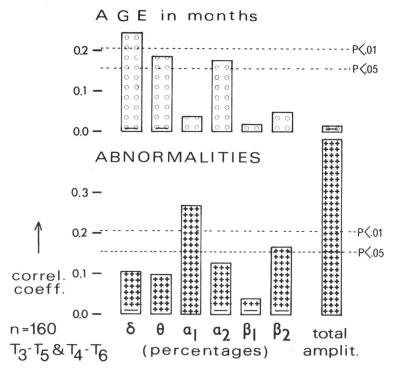

FIG. 8. Correlation of relative amount of EEG activity and the summated amplitudes with
age (upper part) and with visually judged abnormalities in the same recordings (lower part,
N = 15 from the total 160). The sign "—" in the respective column means that the correlation is negative.

2 frequency bands. When compared with the influence of abnormalities, there are quite different relationships between slower and faster alpha activity, as well as between delta and theta activity.

In adolescents some significant changes dependent on sex may be found also (Fig. 9). There is a significantly higher quantity in both beta frequency bands and a slightly lower quantity of delta activity.

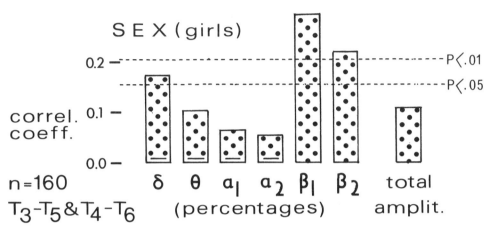

FIG. 9. Correlations between EEG amplitudes and sex. The sign "—" in the respective column means that the correlation is negative; i.e., the amplitude of the respective activity is lower in girls.

No "clinical" item (see Methods) correlates significantly with any of the EEG parameters used, with a few exceptions. In children, the subjects with "sporadic orthostatic collapses" ($N = 67$ from the total 401 individuals) have a very slight increase of alpha 2 activity in frontal derivations (correlation coefficient between the amplitude and occurrence of the symptom 0.109). Similarly, in subjects with "affective lability" ($N = 32$ from 401 individuals), a somewhat higher quantity of theta activity has been found in derivation C0–C3 (correlation coefficient 0.123). In adolescents, a significant correlation appears between the item "head injury without cerebral symptoms" ($N = 5$ from the total 160 individuals) and the amount of theta activity expressed in percentages. The correlation coefficient is 0.225 in fronto-temporal and 0.217 in temporal derivations.

The Effect of Hyperventilation

The amplitudes in all frequency bands increased during hyperventilation. The general effect is somewhat disproportional in different frequency bands, and in different age categories (Fig. 10). There was a clear preference for delta and theta activity in children. Symmetry and variability of EEG activities were not influenced significantly by the activation procedure. The changes of theta/alpha quotient were less prominent than the changes occurring in both frequency bands, if untransformed values were taken into account.

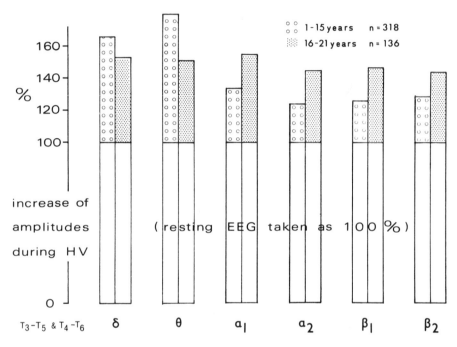

FIG. 10. Effect of hyperventilation. The amplitudes before activation taken as 100%; shown separately are increases in children (circles) and adolescents (dots).

The intensity of hyperventilation was registered by means of subjective criteria. It correlated significantly with the above-mentioned increase of amplitudes, but it did not correlate significantly with age. The correlation between increase of amplitudes and age was significant in most frequency bands, with exception of alpha 1. The respective correlation coefficients were −0.541 for delta, −0.512 for theta, −0.058 for alpha 1, −0.309 for alpha 2, −0.210 for beta 1, and 0.404 for beta 2. All these results concerned children between 1 and 15 years of age. There were no significant correlations in adolescents between the increase of amplitudes and age, with exception of delta activity (correlation coefficient −0.187).

DISCUSSION

The everyday task of electroencephalographers to discriminate between normal and abnormal in the EEG has always called attention to the need of sufficient normative data. Studies on more or less healthy subjects have been provided repeatedly since the 1930's in an effort to define normality in statistical terms. To get quantitative data comparable with the visual evaluation of the recording, the frequency analysis has often been used for these purposes.

It was intended in the present research to sample a sufficiently large group of subjects, fulfilling better than previous studies all criteria for "clinical normality." The method of data processing should be compatible with the method supposedly used for the future quantitative evaluation of the EEG background activity. Therefore, a broad-band analog filtering with subsequent digital processing was used as a most economical procedure. Various untransformed and transformed parameters were computed and mutually compared with regard to their size, variability, and symmetry in various EEG derivations. The quantitative approach with better possibilities of statistical treatment of data might elucidate some problems, but new questions arose.

Age and EEG Frequency Patterns

The dependence of EEG activities on age is well known from the visual evaluation of recordings. By improper treatment of data the quantitative measurement may cause confusion rather than elucidation of facts. For example, owing to general decrease of amplitudes with age, the untransformed quantity of EEG activity and the same expressed percentages may differ from each other. As shown in Table 2 (alpha 1 or beta 1 frequency bands, fronto-temporal derivations, age groups 1–15 years), the quantity may decrease significantly with age, whereas the same value expressed in percentages increases significantly. The question arises which of these seemingly controversial facts is more important for conventional electroencephalography. Usually, the results of frequency analysis are presented as untransformed quantities in scientific publications, since the latter parameters are more closely related to the visual evaluation of the EEG.

Another interesting point is the artificial division of the EEG activities into frequency bands. The frequency analyzer used for this study respects the conventionally accepted bands such as delta and theta. Thus, it is possible to demonstrate various culminating points for different EEG activities at certain ages (Fig. 3). The described points are artificial, however, owing to the generally accepted limits of frequency bands. In fact, there is a continuum from delta frequencies in the youngest age groups to beta frequencies which increase in older individuals. It follows that the mean frequency may serve as a simple but efficient EEG parameter characterizing age-dependent changes of brain activity. This is true at least in children, where the correlation of respective activities with age is relatively high. Owing to increased variability and the weaker influence of the age factor in individuals older than approximately 15 years, some more complicated statistical methods should be applied.

Between 16 and 21 years, the age-dependent changes begin to slow down. Mathematically seen, most of the EEG parameters show logarithmic rather than linear dependency on age. In children the course is more or less linear. The maturation of brain activity is not finished even at 21 years, the upper age limit in this study.

Intra-Individual Variability

Changes of the amplitudes are supposed to be closely related to processing of information in the brain (Walter and Yeager, 1956; Case, 1962; Dubikajtis and Dubikajtis, 1963). The intra-individual "second-to-second" variability corresponds approximately to the visually observable modulation of EEG rhythms. It should be mentioned that the intra-individual variability is of the same order in various age groups, being highest in alpha frequency bands. Only in the youngest age group is the variability somewhat higher in the theta band. More detailed study on intra-individual variability could perhaps contribute to research on biological significance of dominant theta activity in younger children compared with alpha activity in adults. The obtained data are not conclusive where this theoretical question is concerned. The data are satisfactory for another practically important conclusion, however. If the variability of output values is similar in various age groups, no special adjustment of the examination procedure (length of analyzed epochs, for instance) seems to be necessary in younger and older individuals. This fact may simplify the future automation of EEG examinations.

Inter-Individual Variability

Within each age group, a mean amplitude for each frequency component has been stated which enables one to obtain an impression about a most typical frequency pattern for that respective age. The individual values differ from each other in various individuals, however. Information on these deviations from the mean and therefore from the most typical pattern may be had from the inter-individual variability. The lower the variability, the more narrow the normal limits. Because the values obtained in normal and abnormal recordings overlap, the parameters with lower variability are more valuable in the estimation of normality.

In the visual evaluation of routine EEGs, the degree of uncertainty seems to be higher in children than in adults. This fact is usually explained by the increased variability of the EEG in childhood (Hughes, 1961). Surprisingly enough, in our results the inter-individual variability is significantly lower in younger individuals for most parameters used. It means that the frequency pattern of an EEG is more uniform, and any deviation should be more easily detected only in lower age groups. It follows that any uncertainty depends only on inadequacy of methods and does not consist in some unfavorable qualities of the object of observation. It is understandable that even an experienced electroencephalographer simply cannot keep in mind all frequency patterns as they occur in various age groups with sufficient accuracy. Some kind of automatic analysis can avoid such difficulties, if satisfactory normative data do exist.

Topological Aspects

To make the statistical treatment of obtained data easier, some quotients for expressing the symmetry and relationships between anterior and posterior derivations have been used (Fig. 5).

The symmetry ratio correlates significantly with age; the differences between hemispheres are less prominent in younger children and increase in older individuals. The symmetry ratio itself is an interesting EEG parameter which could be used for the estimation of pathological unilateral changes. It is relatively constant in various frequency bands, and its variability is low. From this point of view, the symmetry of theta activity expressed in percentages of the total EEG activity seems to be most advantageous.

It should be noticed that the symmetry is dependent also on the vigilance level: in many parameters a significant decrease of the symmetry ratio has appeared in subjects with drowsiness during the EEG examination (although only EEG samples without any apparent sleep activity have been analyzed).

Differences between EEG activities derived from fronto-temporal and from parieto-occipital leads are considerably greater, and variability of the ratio is relatively high. Its practical application as an EEG parameter serving for further localization of pathological changes is therefore questionable. The ratio decreases significantly with age, which corresponds to increasing differences between mentioned derivations in older individuals.

The quotients used do not elucidate all disproportionalities in age-dependent changes of the EEG activities. Using a parameter with the highest correlation to age, a rapidly proceeding maturation in posterior areas and some delay in frontal and central areas may be demonstrated (Fig. 4). Both decrease of lower frequencies and increase of alpha activity is more pronounced and occurs earlier in posterior derivations (Figs. 1 and 2). This finding may explain some wandering of EEG abnormalities from posterior areas forward, as observed in children during repeated EEG examinations. The maturation process is faster, and therefore, EEG changes related to immaturity of the brain disappear sooner in posterior areas. Besides this, some fictitious shifts may occur because the amplitude of dominating alpha activity increases more rapidly in the posterior derivations. Thus, all EEG events occurring with smaller amplitudes remain hidden among high-voltage alpha waves, being still apparent in anterior areas with smaller amplitude of alpha activity. Also, this hypothesis supports the importance of frequency analysis in children; during analysis, all frequency components are measured more or less independently, which is impossible in visual evaluation of the EEG.

To summarize the topological aspects, the increased variability and amplitude differences in various derivations could be interpreted as EEG correlates of a successive functional differentiation of various brain areas during maturation. Maturation occurs more slowly in frontal and central areas and more rapidly in posterior parts.

Sex Differences

Significant sex differences have been found only among the adolescents. In females, the quantity of beta activity is higher than in males (Fig. 9). Even if some sex differences do exist in younger individuals, they may remain less prominent in comparison with the strongly influential age factor.

The finding of increased amount of beta activity in females between 16 and 21 years of age agrees with the visual evaluation of the same material (Eeg-Olofsson, 1971). The sex differences found in younger subjects and in other frequency bands (Petersén and Eeg-Olofsson, 1971) do not appear in results of frequency analysis, perhaps because of their episodic nature.

In connection with averaging during analysis, the method is less sensitive to transitory events.

Among nonparoxysmal phenomena, higher alpha frequency has been found in girls visually which cannot be confirmed by frequency analysis.

There are several possible explanations: (1) the frequency shifts are so small that the broad-band method is inadequate to detect them; (2) the phenomena described visually are given by some additional episodically occurring activity, whereas the background activity remains unaffected; or (3) owing to the "averaging" of frequencies during the visual evaluation, a mixture of slower beta components with alpha activity may be taken as an equivalent of somewhat higher alpha frequency.

A relative increase of beta activity has already been described in connection with the menstrual cycle (Margerison, Andersson, and Dawson, 1967; Roubíček, Volavka and Matoušek, 1968). In our material, this fact may explain the occurrence of corresponding changes only in older individuals. Some additional factors also cannot be excluded. During the EEG examination a significantly increased anxiety in females has been noticed when compared with that of males of the same age. The amount of beta activity is related to anxiety of the examined subject, which has been found even in normal populations (Volavka et al., 1968). The emotional state may contribute in this way to sex differences among EEG frequency patterns.

Effect of Hyperventilation

The results obtained during hyperventilation should be evaluated cautiously because the intensity of hyperventilation has been estimated only by means of subjective criteria. The reliability of present findings is somewhat supported by the fact that the subjectively registered intensity of hyperventilation does not correlate significantly with age (perhaps owing to selection of proper individuals).

A general increase of amplitude has been noticed in all frequency components and age groups. This increase is more or less proportional in adolescents, since increase in delta and theta frequency bands is more typical for children. In individuals older than 16 years, these changes are relatively independent of age, with the exception of delta activity. In children the hyperventilation effect is strongly affected by the age factor.

For practical purposes it may be of some importance that the symmetry of various EEG activities is not influenced significantly by the activation procedure. No EEG parameter obtained during hyperventilation correlates significantly with normality or abnormality of the EEG, according to visual judgment. On the other hand, there is a significant correlation of the EEG hyperventilation effect and intensity of hyperventilation, in many cases also with the age of examined subject. Thus if the EEG recording during activation does not correlate significantly with asymmetry and abnormality, and if the evoked changes correlate mostly with the intensity of ventilation and with age, then the whole procedure does not contribute significantly to the evaluation of EEG background activity in similar material.

The Question of Normality

In studies dealing with normal populations the question of clinical normality of examined subjects is of primary importance. Studies on adults (Matoušek, Volavka and Roubíček, 1967; Roubíček, Volavka and Matoušek, 1967) have shown that EEG is an extremely sensitive diagnostic tool that reacts to even minimal pathological influences as they may occur in randomly selected subjects without apparent disease states. In this study, relatively strict criteria of normality were used in order to get a better approximation to the hypothetical "ideal" norm. It is quite clear that some factors could remain latent even during a very detailed clinical examination, as pointed out in previously published reports.

As a model of such latent factors, some minimal deviations in the case history have been used (see Methods). There are only a very few significant correlations between some of these items and the EEG amplitudes, the most being debatable "head injury without cerebral symptoms." Among 160 adolescents, five of them answered positively the question about head injury in the past. They denied loss of consciousness and other cerebral symptoms in connection with the trauma.

The correlation coefficient between the occurrence of the item and the percentage of theta activity reaches a significant value of 0.217 in temporal derivations. No significant correlations appear in the other EEG derivations or in other frequency bands. The question arises whether this finding occurs purely at random. (Some coefficients in an extensive correlation matrix may be higher without actual significance, particularly if the number of subjects is small.) On the other hand, it is not possible to exclude the fact that some of these five subjects had suffered from a minute brain injury. Small injuries certainly did occur in many subjects, and it was the subjectively estimated severity which led to a positive answer to the question. It is understandable that no further limits and more detailed objective criteria for excluding the subjects could be applied. Therefore, these sorts of inaccuracies may occur in the material. Much more important seems to be the question of whether it has some practical importance for distortion of obtained data. In the case cited, even in most exposed age group (17 years, with two positive answers from the total 32), the original value for theta activity decreased from 15.86 to 15.72 after omitting the respective two subjects. If the mentioned observation may be taken as representative, then the size of possible resting inaccuracies is even in this extreme case more than negligible (0.9% of the original value). Such an error is much less important than inevitable technical inaccuracies of EEG amplifiers, for instance. To summarize, there are good reasons to consider the present material as sufficient for getting statistical normative data.

Practical Significance of the Present Results

The present study aimed to find out statistical normative data and to contribute in this way to theoretical knowledge on the development of brain activity in human beings. Furthermore, it brought out some data and EEG parameters which could be used in the evaluation of EEG in connection with different pathological states.

As shown, some parameters are more and some are less sensitive to the age factor. To express directly the amount of theta activity, the percentage of theta activity seems to be advantageous, owing to low variability and low age dependency. Whenever the age-dependent changes should be estimated, then the empirical theta (alpha + 8) quotient is most profitable. It correlates in the highest possible degree with the age in all EEG derivations used and age categories (Fig. 7 and Table 2). The quotient concentrates information contained in both theta and alpha frequency bands. It has been found that adding some correcting value to the mean amplitude of alpha activity (in this case the optimum value is "8," the originally suggested somewhat lower value; Matoušek, 1968) increases the significance of the parameter. Another way will be using multivariate statistical methods for choosing a suitable combination of simple parameters which correlates in the highest degree with age.

An interesting and unexpected finding is the decreased inter-individual variability of most EEG parameters in younger individuals. Besides this, the EEG activity is more symmetrical and differences between various EEG derivations in longitudinal direction are less prominent than in older age groups. It means that the children's EEGs are more uniform than the re-cordings in older individuals. With sufficient normative data, the automatic methods of EEG analysis may therefore improve significantly the visual evaluation of background activity, because the age-dependent changes may better separated from other possible deviations. It is especially difficult   ep in mind all frequency patterns as they occur in various age groups.   ficulty disappears if the frequency composition is quantified and com-   e numerically expressed statistical norm. In this way it is pos-   whether the respective EEG curve belongs to the normal   ther way seems to be more advantageous from a practical   in similarities in the frequency composition of abnormal

EEGs and normal recordings in younger individuals can be used for this purpose. It is possible to find out a very similar normal curve belonging to certain age group for any newly examined EEG. The relationship between such a hypothetical and actual age may then serve as a measure of normality or abnormality; the procedure is analogous to the measurement of the IQ. The main advantage would be the ease of evaluating and following all pathological changes in various ages. To a certain extent, the method also allows one mutually to compare results obtained with different methods of EEG analysis. Last but not least the suggested procedure would avoid the well-known difficulties connected with the different subjective criteria of normality of electroencephalographers. Another interesting point is the possible use of frequency analysis for the estimation of maturation defects in EEG. It is hoped that some topological differences as well as the proportionality within the alpha frequency band may be helpful in the discriminating of pathological and normal but immature EEG frequency patterns. Furthermore, longitudinal follow-up studies are in progress, in order to complete the hitherto gained knowledge on normal brain activity in children and adolescents.

SUMMARY

This study deals with EEG findings in normal children (1–16 years) and adolescents (16–22 years) as obtained by means of frequency analysis. The main intention has been to approximate the normative data concerning quite healthy populations as closely as possible. In the study various EEG parameters have been calculated and mutually compared as regards age, sex and other factors. Both the size and topology of EEG changes are demonstrated. The results may be summarized as follows.

1. The data obtained may be taken as representative for a healthy population with sufficient reliability. The estimated resting inaccuracies do not exceed inevitable errors owing to the technical part of EEG examination procedure.

2. Age-dependent changes occurring in various frequency bands have been described quantitatively. Because the total amplitude decreases with age, the absolute and relative changes (e.g., expressed in percentages of the total EEG activity) in the same frequency bands may differ substantially.

3. The development of brain activity proceeds faster in posterior areas and is relatively slower in central areas. In adolescents, all age-dependent changes slow down. The course becomes approximately logarithmic in older age groups, since the dependency on age is almost linear in most EEG parameters as regards younger individuals.

4. Inter-individual variability, asymmetry and differences between activities registered from anterior and posterior derivations tend to increase with age.

5. Intra-individual variability (*i.e.*, fluctuation of amplitudes during the examination) remains similar in various age groups. The variability is somewhat higher in dominant activity when compared with other frequency components.

6. Sex differences: a significantly higher amount of beta activity has been found in girls.

7. During hyperventilation a general increase of amplitudes is more or less proportional in adolescents, since the delta and theta activity preferably increases in children.

8. Some differences between immature and mature but abnormal EEGs have been found. It is possible to diagnose objectively the so-called maturation defect by distinguishing the above-named cases.

9. Among 245 various EEG parameters, a theta/alpha quotient with an empirically stated correction correlates in the highest degree with age, independently of the EEG derivation used and the age category. The use of such a single parameter or optional combination of more parameters for automatic and quantitative evaluation of EEGs has been discussed.

REFERENCES

Bingley, T. (1958): Mental symptoms in temporal lobe gliomas. With special reference to laterality of lesion and the relationship between handedness and brainedness. *Acta Psychiatrica et Neurologica Scandinavica,* Suppl. 120, 151 pp.

Case, T. J. (1962): The clinical significance of changes in the alpha waves. Universitas Medica, 5:27–32.

Dubikajtis, J., and Dubikajtis, V. (1963): The potential field of alpha rhythm on the head surface in human. *Biofizika,* 8:77–81. (*in Russian*)

Eeg-Olofsson, O. (1971): The development of the electroencephalogram in normal adolescents from the age of 16 through 21 years. *Neuropädiatrie,* 3:11–45.

Hughes, R. R. (1961): *An Introduction to Clinical Electro-Encephalography.* John Wright & Sons Ltd., Bristol, 118 pp.

Kaiser, E., Petersén, I., Selldén, U., and Kagawa, N. (1964): EEG data representation in broad-band frequency analysis. *Electroencephalography and Clinical N---*

Petersén, I., and Eeg-Olofsson, O. (1970/71): The development of the electroencephalogram in normal children from the age of 1 through 15 years. Non-paroxysmal activity. *Neuropädiatrie*, 2:247–304.

Petersén, I., Eeg-Olofsson, O., Hagne, I., and Selldén, U. (1965): EEG of selected healthy children. *Electroencephalography and Clinical Neurophysiology*, 19:613–620.

Petersén, I., Eeg-Olofsson, O., and Selldén, U. (1968): Paroxysmal activity in EEG of normal children. In: *Clinical Electroencephalography of Children*, edited by P. Kellaway and I. Petersén. Almqvist & Wiksell, Stockholm, pp. 167–187.

Petersén, I., and Matoušek, M. (1972): Breitband-Frequenz Analyse der Elektroenzephalogramme bei normalen Kindern und Jugendlichen. *EEG-EMG* (Stuttgart), 3:134–138.

Roubíček, J., Tachezy, R., and Matousek, M. (1968): Electric activity of the brain in the course of menstrual cycle. *Československa Psychiatrie*, 64:90–94. (*in Czech.*)

Roubíček, J., Volavka, J., and Matoušek, M. (1967): EEG in normal population. II: Physiological changes and EEG. *Ceskoslovenska Psychiatrie*, 63:14–19. (*in Czech.*)

Volavka, J., Matoušek, M., and Roubíček, J. (1968): EEG frequency analysis and neurotic symptoms in normal population. *Bratislavske Lekarske Listy*, 49:659–664. (*in Czech.*)

Walter, R. D., and Yeager, C. L. (1956): Visual imagery and electroencephalographic changes. *Electroencephalography and Clinical Neurophysiology*, 8:193–199.

Automation of Clinical Electroencephalography.
Edited by P. Kellaway and I. Petersén.
Raven Press, New York © 1973.

Spectral Analysis via Fast Fourier Transform of Waking EEG in Normal Infants

I. Hagne, J. Persson, R. Magnusson and I. Petersén

Department of Clinical Neurophysiology, Sahlgrenska Sjukhuset, Göteborg; Department of Pediatrics, University of Göteborg, Departments of Electrical Measurements and Applied Electronics, Chalmers University of Technology, Göteborg, Sweden

The first year of life is a period of very rapid physical and mental development. There are also rapid changes in the electroencephalogram. With the exception of the neonatal period, infants have been subject to relatively little attention in the EEG literature, especially regarding the maturation process in normal children. The shortage of normative data has limited the usefulness of EEG as a tool for diagnosis and prognosis in this age group, in which the need for such tools is especially great.

The need for quantitative methods for description of the EEGs development during childhood was reflected in the very first works on the subject (Lindsley, 1938, 1939; Bernhard and Skoglund, 1939; Henry, 1944). Manual measurements were then made of frequencies and amplitudes, and the results were presented as mean values or indices. In this manner, such data as the frequency development of dominant activity and the relative share of alpha and delta activity in the trace at various ages could be described. Manual frequency analysis was also subsequently used on a child material by Fujimori, Yokota, Ishibashi, and Takel (1958) in a comparative
different method

old children, the latter author found in a manual count of frequency distribution in the awake EEG that inter-individual variations were very great with respect to the dominant frequency. He regarded the theta-alpha mean value (TAM) as a better measure of EEG development at this age than dominant frequency. However, manual methods of analysis are time consuming and provide relatively little information.

Data on normal child EEGs processed with automatic frequency analysis were published in a preliminary form by Knott and Gibbs as early as 1939 and in greater detail by Gibbs and Knott (1949). There were 37 term newborns or older infants in the study. The major part of the activity in this age group was found to be concentrated in the low frequency part of the spectrum and that up to the age of 1 year, only "the shoulder of the low frequency peak" reached 9 Hz. Grey Walter (1950) concluded on the basis of his own frequency analysis of the child EEG that delta activity dominates up to the age of 1 year, and that it is usually diffuse and often asymmetrical. There was an alpha rhythm even in the youngest age group which, however, displayed certain differences compared to adult alpha activity. "Extreme variability" was found by this author in all age groups. Corbin and Bickford (1955), who made a comparison between visual evaluation and automatic frequency analysis of child EEGs, also found great variability among different individuals but great consistency of pattern in the individual recordings. The agreement between homologous regions in the two hemispheres of the same child was "remarkably close." One of the illustrations in their report shows that the mean spectrum in the parieto-occipital region for 1-year-olds was limited to the delta and theta regions and that there was no distinct frequency peak; there was, however, a "hump" at 5–6 Hz. Only eight infants (1-year-olds) were included in this study. Fujimori, Yokota, Ishibashi, and Takel (1958) performed automatic frequency analysis (Offner analyzer), mathematical analysis (manual Fourier transform) and amplitude histograms on a material made up of 43 normal children, 3 months to 14 years old. Detailed results of the EEG analyses from different age groups were not reported. The emphasis of the article was on a comparison of the three methods used. Frequency analysis of the EEGs of normal children of varying ages and with different techniques was also performed by Drohocki and Duflo (1958), Hashimoto and Hamava (1963), Gabersek and Scherrer (1966), Arakawa, Mizuno, Chiba, Sakai, Watanabe, and Tamura, (1968), Rémond, Lesèvre, Joseph, Rieger, and Lairy, (1969), Lairy, Rémond, Rieger, and Lesèvre, (1969), Matoušek and Petersén (this volume). Infants were involved only to a limited extent or not at all in these reports.

The frequency analysis work performed on infants has usually dealt with the neonatal period (Bartoshuk, 1964; Nolte, Schulte, Michaelis, and Juergens, 1968; Nolte, Schulte, Michaelis, Weisse, and Gruson, 1969; Prechtl, 1968; Prechtl, Weinmann, and Akiyama, 1969; Schulte, Hinze, and Schrempf, 1971). In these cases EEG was recorded as part of a polygraphic investigation of the spontaneous course of sleep. In certain cases, pathological groups were compared with small groups of normal cases or "control cases." In a few studies frequency analysis was performed on a longitudinal infant material during sleep (Parmelee, Akiyama, Schultz, Wenner and Schulte, 1969) and during wakefulness (Mizuno, Yamauchi, Watanabe, Komatsushiro, Takagi, Iinuma, and Arakawa, 1970). Mizuno examined a group of 10 normal infants once a month during the first year of life. He used a frequency analyzer with 10 frequency bands and presented his results in the form of peak frequencies and as ratios between activities in two groups of compounded frequency bands, individually and as mean values for different age groups. An illustration of the mean spectrum at 3, 6 and 12 months discloses no obvious frequency peaks, but there is a certain displacement of the spectrum's main energy toward higher frequencies as age increases. Because of the small samples in each age group, no general conclusions can be drawn from this material.

Most of the materials mentioned above were analyzed with analog instruments. However, numerical spectral analysis with a computer was performed in a number of cases generally via autocorrelation (Prechtl, 1968; Prechtl, Weinmann and Akiyama, 1969; Parmelee, Akiyama, Schultz, Wenner and Schulte, 1969; Schulte, Hinze and Schrempf, 1971). In a spectral analysis study of twins, Dumermuth (1968, 1969) performed Fast Fourier Transform (FFT) according to the method introduced by Cooley and Tukey in 1965. Dumermuth (1971) has also published a survey of computer analysis of children's EEGs and has recently given a comprehensive presentation of methods for spectral analysis of EEG (*in press*).

In a previous publication, Hagne (1968) described the development of the awake EEG during the first year of life in a group of healthy children selected according to strict criteria. The children were subjected to longitudinal follow-up from birth with EEGs, neurological examinations and psychometric development evaluation. The report published the results of visual evaluation and frequency analysis with broadband filters of the awake EEG. In recent years, new methods of analysis have been developed with which further information could conceivably be elicited from the taped records. One such method, spectral analysis via FFT, has now been applied to the

MATERIAL

The material of the present investigation comprises awake recordings of the same longitudinal, healthy-infant material which has previously been described in detail (Hagne, 1968). All the children were also followed after the age of 1 year and were found at the latest examination – at the age of $3\frac{1}{2}$–6 years – to be neurologically healthy and normally developed. From the total number of 29 infants, only those who produced a minimum of five technically satisfactory awake recordings between the age of 3 weeks to 12 months were included for spectral analysis. In this manner the group came to comprise 20 children. The distribution of the material by age groups is shown in Table 1. In cases satisfying the demand for five technically acceptable waking recordings, one or more leads in a recording occasionally had to be excluded from analysis, however, because artifacts in the trace caused missing values in individual channels and ages. Table 2 shows 599 frequency spectra, distributed by age and lead, which were obtained.

TABLE 1. Number of examinations in each age group

		Frequency analysis	
Age (months)	Awake EEG ($N = 29$)	Broadband ($N = 20$)	FFT ($N = 20$)
$\frac{3}{4}$	22	16	16
2	29	19	19
4	28	18	17
6	28	17	17
8	28	17	17
10	29	17	17
12	26	17	17

N = total number of individuals examined.

TABLE 2. Number of spectra

Lead	Age (months)							Total
	$\frac{3}{4}$	2	4	6	8	10	12	
T_3–T_5	16	18	13	10	10	13	13	93
T_4–T_6	15	16	9	9	11	14	11	85
P_3–O_1	15	15	14	12	15	15	14	100
P_4–O_2	13	16	14	14	13	12	14	96
C_3–C_0	14	19	17	16	17	16	16	115
C_4–C_0	14	16	15	16	16	16	17	110
	87	100	82	77	82	86	85	599

METHODS

EEG Recording

The recordings were made with a 16-channel Kaiser electroencephalograph. The children had open eyes during awake recordings, and they were observed continuously by a specially detached person with respect to movements, sucking, and eye closing in order to obtain the most accurate evaluation possible of the "state" and identification of movement artifacts. Electrode placement was according to the 10/20 system. Bipolar leads were used according to Fig. 1. The time constant was 0.3 sec, and the recorder was calibrated to make 5 mm correspond to 50 μV peak to peak. In addition to EEG, eye movements and the EKG were also recorded.

A tape recording was made, at the same time as the conventional EEG recording, from six pairs of electrodes for subsequent automatic frequency analysis of a temporal, a parieto-occipital and a central lead from each hemisphere (Fig. 1). Frontal leads were not analyzed because of eye movements and blink artifacts in these leads. Sixty-sec (exceptionally 50 or 40 sec) epochs, free or nearly free from artifacts, were chosen for frequency

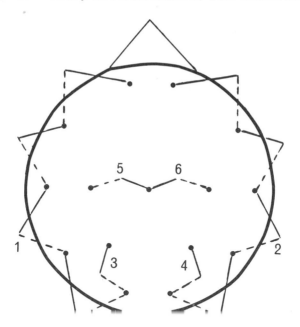

analysis. Since, as a rule, awake babies never lie still very long, it often was necessary to select two or more separate epochs in order to obtain a technically acceptable recording lasting a total of 60 sec.

Spectral Analysis

The Measurement System. A block diagram of the measurement system is shown in Fig. 2. The EEGs were recorded on magnetic tape at the same time as paper registration. For calibration purposes, each EEG record was preceded by a set of sine waves of frequencies 2.2, 4.8, 8.2, 10.9, 15.2 and 21.6 Hz and amplitudes of 50 μV peak to peak. The calibration signals were originally chosen to suit a broadband analyzer and mainly intended to equalize the gain of the different channels. Their accuracy was low, which implies a low accuracy in estimated absolute power densities of the EEGs.

Besides, since there are no calibration signals below 2.2 Hz, this part of the amplitude characteristic had to be roughly estimated with subsequent uncertainty of the spectral slopes in this range (Persson, 1971). Steps P2–P4 in Fig. 2 were introduced because of the need to edit the tape, thus providing it with a command signal, yielding start and stop pulses for computer input. In order to arrive at a simple calibration of the power spectrum, a noise generator of known power density was inserted at point P3. The EEG signal was entered into a low pass filter with a cut-off frequency of 42 Hz and a damping rate of 24 dB/octave above this frequency. The analog signal was digitized at a frequency of 102.4 Hz, which yields negligible aliasing effects in the frequency band studied, 1.0–12.8 Hz (see below). The spectra were calculated on an IBM 1800 computer by means of an FFT algorithm for real valued series (Bergland 1969).

Spectral Estimation. In most cases, records of 60-sec duration were used for the calculation of a spectrum. Because of the computer's limited core-memory capacity (24 k), the records were divided into 10-sec segments. The average of the calculated segment periodograms[1] for one record was taken as a record spectrum.

The variability of the spectral estimator was reduced by the use of segments having a 50% overlap in time, as shown in Fig. 3. Each segment data sample was multiplied by a data window of shape $(1 - t^2)$, as illustrated in Fig. 4. This procedure yields a reduction in the interference between different frequency bands. Thus, in this case the side lobes of the spectral window fall off at a rate of -12 dB/octave, whereas the corresponding rate in the rectangular data window case is -6 dB/octave.

---

[1] The periodogram is the square of the absolute value of the Fourier transform of a data sample.

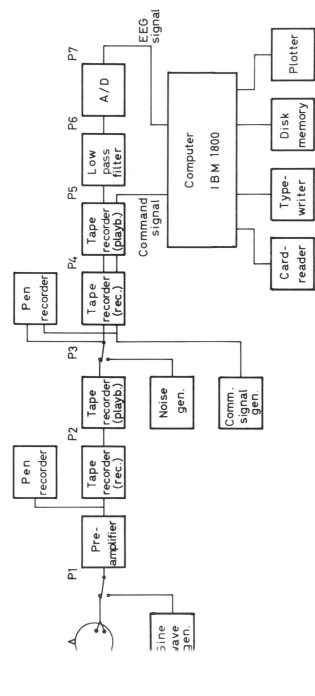

2. Block diagram of the measurement system.

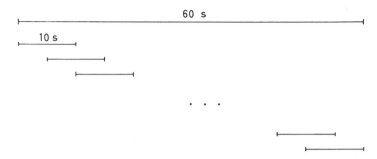

FIG. 3. Segmentation of one EEG record of 60-sec. length.

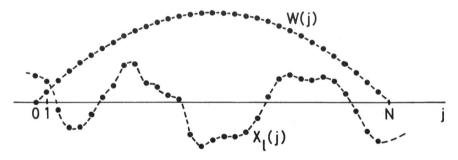

FIG. 4. Sampled EEG segment $X_l(j)$ and data window $W(j)$.

The record spectra thus derived were further smoothed by forming a weighted sum of adjacent spectral values, chosen to give a desired shape and width to the spectral window. In our processing, the shape was approximately triangular, and the half-power width was approximately 0.4 Hz. The envelope of the spectral window is shown in Fig. 5.

The frequency range of special interest was expected to be the delta and theta bands. The analyses were performed and displayed in the range from 1 to 25 Hz. The results showed a remarkable development of activity in the expected range, which led us to carry out a detailed study between 1.0 and 12.8 Hz. Above this range, the power densities were rather uniform and of a low level.

Each spectrum was normalized to the average from 1 to 25 Hz. This level corresponds to 0 dB in the plots.

Expressions of the expectation of the spectral estimator and the spectral window are given in the Appendix. In addition, the variability and confidence limits of the spectral estimator in the case of a Gaussian EEG signal are derived.

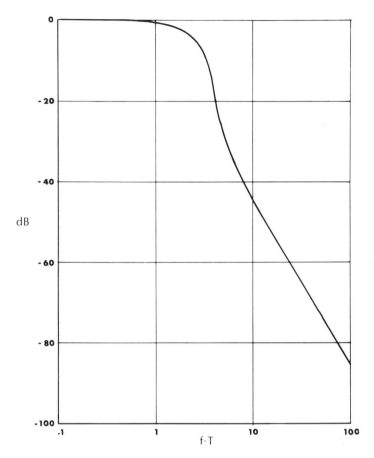

FIG. 5. Envelope of spectral window used.

Peak Detection. In the course of our investigations of infant EEGs, we found a strong noise component of approximately $1/f^2$ frequency dependence. In order to facilitate peak detection and to provide a distinct measure of peak height, the $1/f^2$ component was eliminated by subtracting from the spectrum a least-squares regression line in logarithmic intensity and frequency scales. This regression line was fitted to the spectrum over the range from 1.0 to 12.8 Hz. The remaining spectrum factor, illustrated in Fig. 6, was investigated with regard to spectral peaks.

An empirical study of the results showed that spectral variations, which

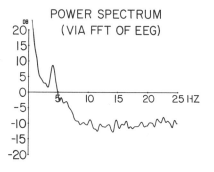 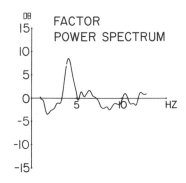

FIG. 6. Factorization of EEG spectrum. (a) Original spectrum. (b) Rippling factor of the spectrum.

for the spectrum in the case of a Gaussian signal, which is derived in the Appendix, peaks greater than 2 dB in the spectrum factor were selected as peaks. The largest peak was subjected to a detailed study concerning appearance, frequency and height. The second peak—if present—and the total spectrum were also investigated.

Statistics

Statistical significances were evaluated at the 5% level.

RESULTS

Since the spectral characteristics of the EEG from the left and the right hemispheres displayed only minor differences (see below), results will be reported here principally for the left hemisphere.

Mean Spectra

A study of the absolute levels of the spectra was generally considered to be of limited value because of the rather poor accuracy in the calibration signal and the attendant uncertainty in absolute spectral values. Following normalization and transformation to the decibel scales, as described under Methods, spectral curves were obtained whose general appearance is shown in Fig. 7. The mean spectrum and standard deviation in the different age groups is shown there for channels T3–T5, P3–O1 and C3–C0.

Means (M) and standard deviations (SD) were calculated with a linear power scale and plotted after transformation to the logarithmic dB scale.

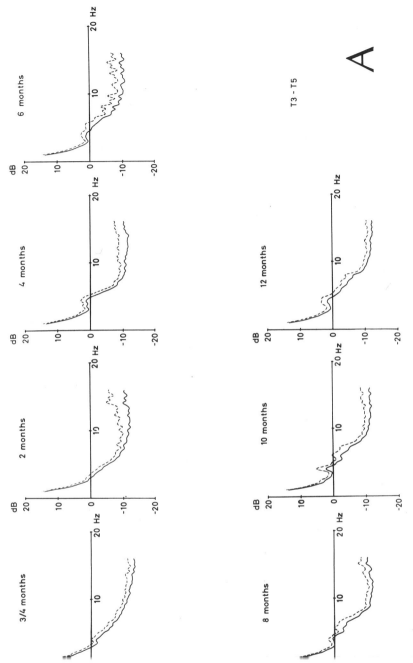

7. Mean and one standard deviation of frequency spectra in the seven age groups studied. Abscissa: frequency in Hz. Ordinate: sity in dB. A: T_3-T_5. B: P_3-O_1. C: C_3-C_0.

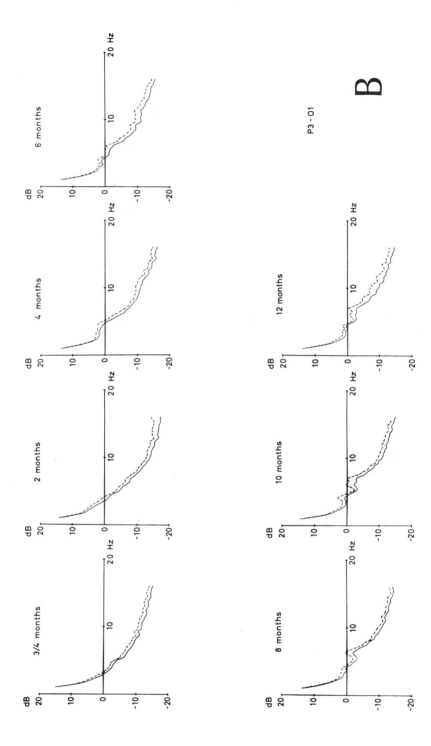

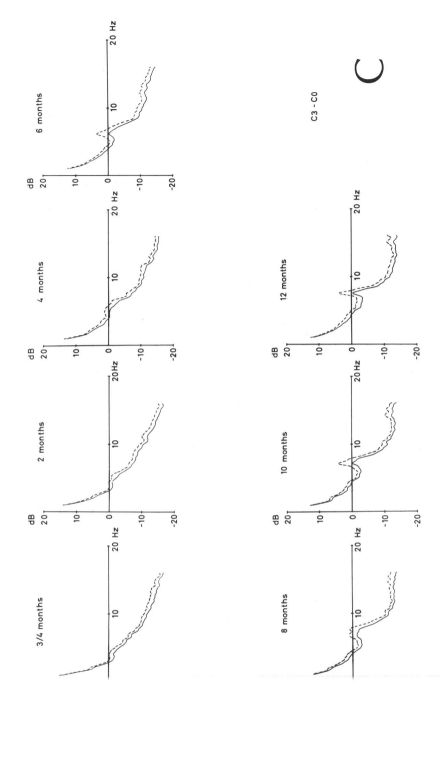

Thus, the mean is represented by $10 \log_{10} M$ and the variability by $10 \log_{10} (M + SD)$, giving a distance between the two curves corresponding to $10 \log_{10} (1 + SD/M)$. As seen in Fig. 7, this distance, except for the peak region, is rather uniform and approximately 1–2 dB, which corresponds to a coefficient of variation (SD/M) of approximately 0.3–0.6.

As is also seen, activity is concentrated to the delta-theta region during the whole first year. For the lower age groups, the spectra decrease rather smoothly from low to high frequencies. From 4 to 6 months of age, more or less obvious peaks arise within the theta region.

The variability is generally higher in the peak region, which is sometimes quite diffuse. Occasionally, even double peaks appear.

Only the range from 1.0 to 12.8 Hz was included in the continued processing of the spectra, since the activity level in the frequency range beyond this region was very low and was occasionally influenced by muscle potentials. A measure of the distribution of intensity between fast and slow spectral components is provided by the *slope* of the spectral curve. The spectral slope, defined as the slope of the regression line fitted to the spectrum in the interval from 1.0 to 12.8 Hz, was studied in order to obtain a general outline of the intensity distribution in this frequency range. Development during the period studied was expressed in all leads by a successively less negative slope, i.e., a reduction in the low-frequency component and an increase in the high-frequency component. The greatest changes are seen in the parieto-occipital leads. Figure 8 shows the mean and standard deviations for the slope expressed in dB/octave. As the figure shows, the standard deviations are large, i.e., of the same magnitude or larger than the change in the slope from one age group to another. The initial dip in lead P3–O1 is not significant (by the *t*-test of differences).

In the mean spectra for the three aforementioned cortical regions (Fig. 7), a hump appears in the temporal and parieto-occipital leads in the 3–5 Hz frequency range at the age of 4 months. This hump then develops into a more or less sharp frequency peak which is successively displaced toward higher frequencies as age increases. The central lead deviates from the other two leads by the hint of a frequency peak detectable as early as 3 weeks of age. The frequency peaks in this lead are also generally more distinct and of higher frequency than those in the parieto-occipital and temporal leads.

Individual Spectra

In individual spectra, a dominant frequency is often much more prominent than in mean spectra. The development of the spectrum in an individual case is illustrated in Fig. 9. Spectra for the same individual at different ages have been drawn into the same figure with an upward displacement of the origin

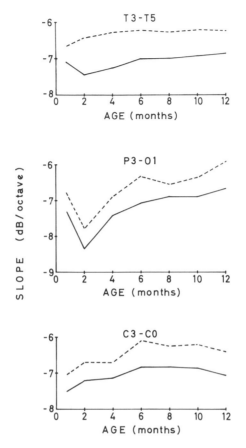

FIG. 8. Mean and one standard deviation of slopes of the spectral curves in three cortical areas during the first year.

of the decibel scale for each age. In this manner the migration of the frequency peak from lower to higher frequencies with increasing age is more clearly illustrated. The peaks in the frequency range from 1.0 to 12.8 Hz which satisfy the criterion for a peak, *i.e.*, a magnitude of at least 2 dB after the factorization described in the section on Methods, are marked with arrows. If, in addition to the dominant peak (solid arrow), one or more peaks satisfying the established criterion occur in the same spectrum, these secondary peaks are marked with dashed arrows. The most regular development of the dominant frequency is seen in the central region where peak frequency

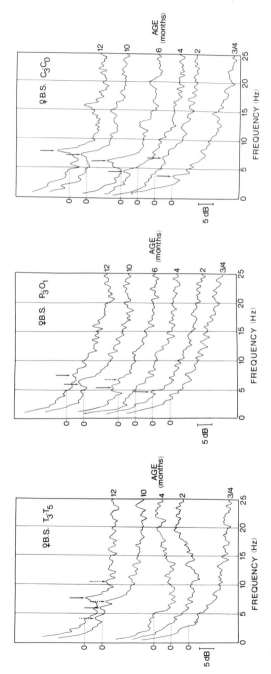

FIG. 9. Development of frequency peaks in one infant from $3/4$–12 months of age in three cortical areas. Solid arrows indicate dominant peak, dashed arrows secondary peaks.

peak is just above the limit chosen for a peak. Development in the other two leads in the same figure is principally the same but somewhat more complex, particularly in the temporal region. There were no peaks at all in this lead up to the age of 4 months. At 10 and 12 months, there were 2 and 1 secondary peaks, respectively, alongside the dominant frequency. Some of the peaks, which are seen above the 12.8 Hz frequency region, consisted of harmonics, e.g., in trace C, 12 months at 16 Hz.

Spectral Peaks

The distribution of the dominant frequency in the entire material is shown in Fig. 10, in which all peak frequency values are plotted versus age, and least squares regression lines are drawn. The steepest curve is seen in P3–O1 and the flattest in T3–T5. C3–C0 has the highest intercept. The spread among individuals in the same age groups was often very wide. Boys and girls are indicated with different symbols. Boys seem to display a tendency to lower peak frequencies than girls. The differences, however, were not statistically significant (by the rank sum test at age 12 months).

Development of the dominant frequency in the individual child was studied in an analogous manner (Fig. 11A–C). A minimum of three observations, including at least one each in the periods from $\frac{3}{4}$ to 4 months and from 8 to 12 months, was stipulated as required to draw a regression line for each lead. The most common appearance, which occurred in approximately 60% of the children, is illustrated in Fig. 11A. The regression there has a similar, ascending course in all three leads. Considerable deviations from this picture could occur, however, as in Fig. 11B, in which the regression line for T3–T5 displays a slightly negative slope, whereas the slope in the other two lines is positive. Figure 11C shows two very irregular developmental patterns for the dominant frequency, with widely scattered values and a negative slope (central lead) in the first case, and initially a descending and then an ascending series of values (parieto-occipital) in the second case.

Peak height is a measure of amplitude and constancy of the dominant frequency. By definition, the lower limit for a peak was 2 dB. The range of variation extended up to 14.8 dB. The mean value in all regions increased from just over 2 dB at 3 weeks to a maximum value at 10–12 months of 6.2 dB centrally, 5.1 dB in the temporal lead and 4.6 dB in the parieto-occipital lead (Table 4, *below*). The spread among individuals was very great, and the variation in the same individual could also be very great between two examination sessions. In some individuals a maximum was reached at the

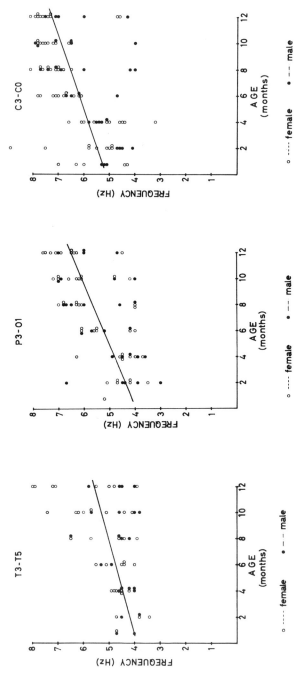

FIG. 10. Peak frequency as a function of age for lead T_3–T_5, P_3–O_1, C_3–C_0, and regression lines fitted to the set of points.

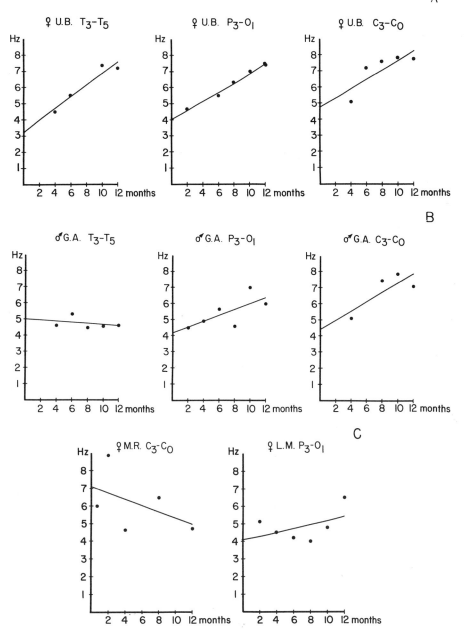

FIG. 11. Individual development of peak frequency. A: Commonest type: upward course of regression line in all leads. ̇ ommon variation: slightly downward course in one lead

TABLE 3. Peak frequency (in Hertz units) for different leads and ages

Age (months)		T_3-T_5	T_4-T_6	P_3-O_1	P_4-O_2	C_3-C_0	C_4-C_0
0.75	M	4.5	4.7	5.2	4.2	5.5	5.6
	SD	0.40	0.14	–	0.92	0.93	0.77
	N	3	2	1	2	8	8
2	M	4.0	4.4	4.4	3.9	5.5	5.1
	SD	0.54	1.57	0.95	0.80	1.33	0.45
	N	5	7	11	7	13	11
4	M	4.4	4.2	4.4	4.2	5.2	5.5
	SD	0.31	0.17	0.71	0.46	0.83	0.79
	N	11	5	12	12	15	13
6	M	4.8	4.8	5.3	5.3	6.7	6.1
	SD	0.52	0.73	0.80	1.04	0.77	1.32
	N	8	7	11	14	14	16
8	M	5.0	5.4	5.8	5.9	6.8	7.0
	SD	0.99	1.18	1.13	0.84	1.13	0.75
	N	9	10	14	12	17	15
10	M	5.3	5.3	6.0	6.2	7.1	7.1
	SD	1.12	1.15	1.11	1.09	0.98	0.94
	N	12	12	14	11	15	16
12	M	5.7	5.6	6.5	6.6	6.9	7.2
	SD	1.49	1.31	0.94	1.01	1.26	1.18
	N	12	11	14	13	16	17

M = mean; SD = standard deviation; N = sample size.

frequency peaks, peak height and peak frequency as a function of age, one picture for each cortical region studied. Except for small deviations, an increase in the percentage of peaks, peak height and peak frequency are seen in all regions as age increases. In all respects the central region is on a higher level than the other two leads and displays a smoother increase. The values for T3–T5 and P3–O1 in the two youngest age groups are rather uncertain because of the small sample size in these cases (see Tables 3 and 4).

Regional Differences

In all age groups there was a considerable loss of values owing to lack of registration, exclusion of one or more leads from the frequency analysis because of artifacts, or to absence of peaks in the spectrum. For that reason the sample in each age and lead is often small and does not comprise exactly the same individuals. On this account a statistical analysis of peak frequency and peak height, including tests of significance of regional and interhemispheric differences, was not possible. In Tables 3 and 4, however,

TABLE 4. Peak height (in decibels) for different leads and ages

Age (months)		T_3-T_5	T_4-T_6	P_3-O_1	P_4-O_2	C_3-C_0	C_4-C_0
0.75	M	2.4	2.5	2.3	2.4	2.9	3.1
	SD	0.26	0.28	–	0.14	0.73	0.46
	N	3	2	1	2	8	8
2	M	2.8	3.2	3.0	3.0	3.2	2.9
	SD	0.38	1.35	0.60	0.53	0.84	0.58
	N	5	7	11	7	13	11
4	M	4.6	3.2	3.8	4.2	4.2	4.1
	SD	1.29	0.80	1.22	1.62	1.34	1.23
	N	11	5	12	12	15	13
6	M	4.5	4.3	4.0	4.0	5.2	4.7
	SD	1.60	1.43	1.20	1.07	2.41	1.97
	N	8	7	11	14	14	16
8	M	4.0	4.2	4.0	3.9	5.5	5.5
	SD	1.38	1.16	1.62	1.90	2.47	2.27
	N	9	10	14	12	17	15
10	M	4.9	4.3	4.2	4.6	6.1	6.2
	SD	2.27	1.86	1.89	2.19	3.01	2.90
	N	12	12	14	11	15	16
12	M	5.1	4.0	3.9	3.9	5.9	5.5
	SD	1.39	1.55	1.79	1.09	3.13	2.60
	N	12	11	14	13	16	17

M = mean; SD = standard deviation; N = sample size.

means and standard deviations are given for the six leads analyzed in each age group. As was obvious from Fig. 12, the central lead generally has higher values of peak frequency than the other two cortical regions, and the parieto-occipital lead in most ages exceeds the temporal lead in this respect. Also regarding peak height, the central leads deviate from the two others by a tendency to display higher values, at least during the second half-year.

As to differences between homologous areas in the two hemispheres, the mean values as a rule agree fairly well for both peak frequency and peak height. No tendency toward a preponderance of one hemisphere regarding these variables can be traced. In individuals, however, there were sometimes considerable interhemispheric differences of peak height or peak frequency.

Differences between cortical regions with respect to absolute mean intensity ($\mu V^2/Hz$) in the range 1–25 Hz were tested by means of analyses of

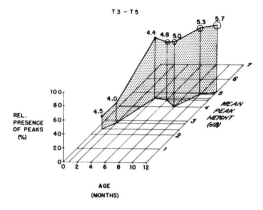

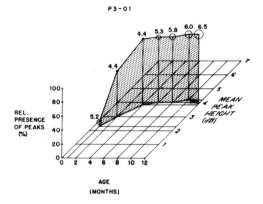

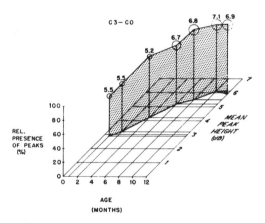

FIG. 12. Relative presence of peaks, mean peak height and mean peak frequency as function of age. The mean peak frequencies are indicated in Hz above circles, whose diameters are proportional to the frequency.

no effect on differences between leads. It is thus justified to use absolute values in this comparison. Only two significant differences were found, *viz.*, for age 2 months between the right temporal and parieto-occipital leads and between the latter lead and the left central lead. Because of missing data, each analysis of variance comprised, however, rather few (from 5 to 12) individuals.

Comparison with Broadband Analyses

A comparison of the results of spectral analysis with the broadband analysis previously performed is possible to a limited extent only. As mentioned above, the absolute values obtained in spectral analysis were generally not used in the statistical processing of data. In some cases the absolute level in the FFT spectrum, expressed in $\mu V^2/Hz$, for the frequency range 1.0–12.8 Hz was compared with the corresponding value from broadband analysis, converted to the same unit, in order to obtain an idea of the relationship between FFT spectral analysis data and the results of broadband analysis. The difference between the two measurement methods amounted to at most 25%. This difference can be explained by the uncertainty of the measurement system's characteristics with respect to low frequencies (below the lowest calibration frequency of 2.2 Hz). A delta/theta ratio was used in the broadband analysis as the unit in the description of frequency development; this ratio, generally speaking, declined with advancing age (Fig. 13). The slope of the spectral curve, where the development curve has a similar but ascending course (Fig. 8), is to some extent an equivalent parameter in spectral analysis. Both methods describe the displacement of the spectrum's main energy from lower to higher frequencies. The delta-theta ratio, however, is derived from the spectrum in the range 1.5–7.5 Hz, whereas for the slope in Fig. 8, the corresponding range is 1.0–12.8 Hz. Frequency peaks in spectral analysis have no equivalent in broadband analysis.

Comparison with Visual Analyses

In the visual evaluation performed in conjunction with broadband analysis, the presence of a dominant activity was determined. If such activity was found to exist, its frequency was estimated. The relative incidence of a peak frequency in visual evaluation and in spectral analysis, respectively, was plotted in Fig. 14. The differences which occurred were most pronounced in the first half-year of life with a tendency to a higher incidence in visual eval-

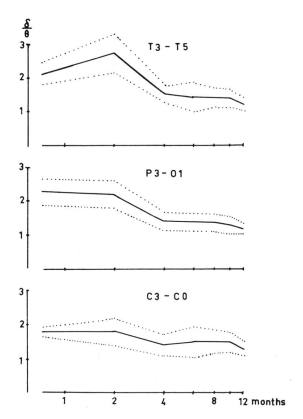

FIG. 13. Means and one standard deviation of ratios delta/theta in broadband analysis as a function of age (logarithmic scale of age).

and automatic evaluation which lacked a dominant activity, even in the oldest age groups.

The values for dominant frequency obtained in visual evaluation and in spectral analysis are compared in Fig. 15, and mean values and standard deviations are stated for both methods. The mean values generally agree rather well, but in some ages and leads the mean value was higher in spectral analysis than in visual evaluation, e.g., in lead C3–C0 at age 6 months. The difference, however, was not statistically significant (by the *t*-test of differences). The spread was consistently greater in spectral analysis than in visual evaluation.

The discrepancy between peak frequency in FFT and visually evaluated dominant activity could be great (up to 3.4 Hz) in individual spectra. Starting with cases in which the difference was more than or equal to 1 Hz, the

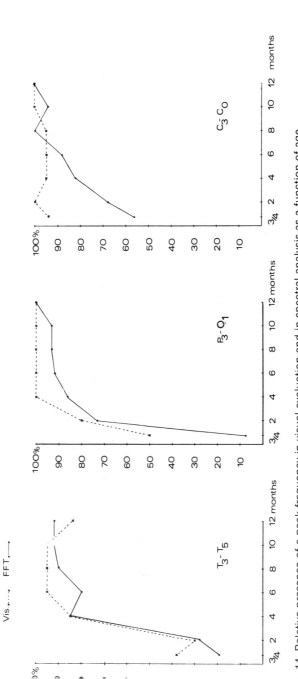

14. Relative presence of a peak frequency in visual evaluation and in spectral analysis as a function of age.

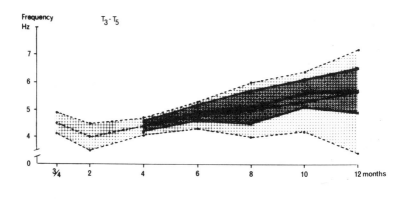

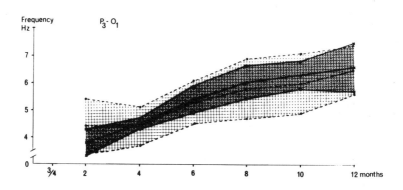

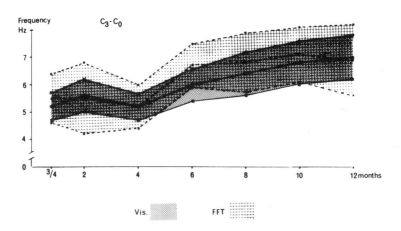

FIG. 15. Mean and one standard deviation of dominant frequency in visual and automatic evaluation. Abscissa: age in months. Ordinate: dominant frequency (Hz).

spectra were further scrutinized. There were 61 such cases, 25 of which with differences greater than or equal to 1.5 Hz. In this new examination of the spectra, we found a further peak, which satisfied the criterion for a peak, in the spectral curve of 17 cases, this secondary peak corresponding to the value for the visual dominant frequency. In 31 cases it was found that the shape of the peak in FFT was broad and occasionally askew. The visual peak lay within another part of this broad "peak" or "hump" than the FFT peak value. In the 13 remaining cases, reexamination of the original EEG traces occasionally disclosed a frequency component corresponding to the FFT value but of a very modest amplitude (10–15 μV). An example is shown in Fig. 16 (right part A and B). In lead C3–C0, the dominant frequency was visually evaluated as 4.5 Hz (most apparent in the lower picture); the peak frequency in FFT was 8.9 Hz. The latter component appears in the upper picture but is not very conspicuous because of the small amplitude. Another reason for the discrepancies between the two methods for determination of the dominating frequency is seen in the left part of Fig. 16. The lower picture, which was part of the frequency analysis, had no spectral peak in channel 3, i.e., the left parieto-occipital lead, and hardly any rhythmic activity is found visually. In the same channel in the upper picture, there is a clear 5–6 Hz rhythm which was visually interpreted as dominant activity. However, this part of the trace was not included in the frequency analysis because of an abundance of artifacts.

In addition to a comparison of the individual parameters in the EEG in visual evaluation and spectral analysis, respectively, it is of interest to establish if spectral analysis can provide an equivalent to the overall picture offered by visual evaluation. The latter procedure comprises not only an estimation of frequency and amplitude of the dominant activity, but also evaluation of such factors as curve regularity, amount of low frequency activity, and rhythms other than the background activity. An idea of the general frequency distribution in a record is obtained from the slope of the spectral curve in combination with the value for one or possibly more peak frequencies. In the previous description of frequency distribution in the EEG in the first year of life (Hagne, 1968), it was pointed out that the individual child usually retains a given character of the EEG throughout this period with respect to frequency composition, a "slow" type in some cases, a "fast" type in others. Fig. 17 shows the development in two children of such extreme types of EEG as manifest at three different ages in the conventional EEG record, the left being "slow" and the right "fast." If the regression lines for the development of peak frequency in spectral analysis from

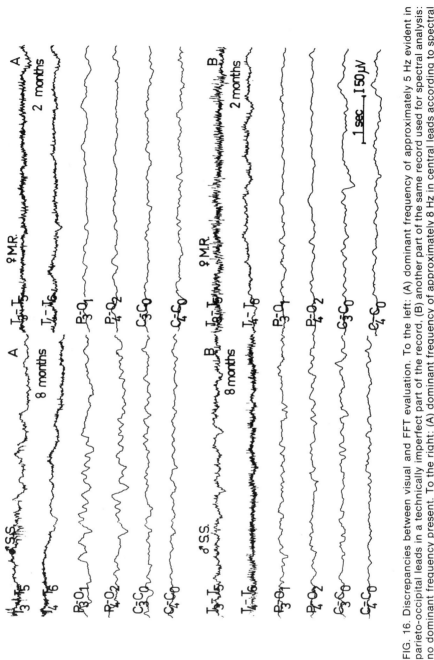

FIG. 16. Discrepancies between visual and FFT evaluation. To the left: (A) dominant frequency of approximately 5 Hz evident in parieto-occipital leads in a technically imperfect part of the record, (B) another part of the same record used for spectral analysis: no dominant frequency present. To the right: (A) dominant frequency of approximately 8 Hz in central leads according to spectral analysis; same frequency hardly visible in the written record due to small amplitude, (B) visual evaluation of the same leads: "dominant" frequency 4.5 Hz, appearing in short sequences only.

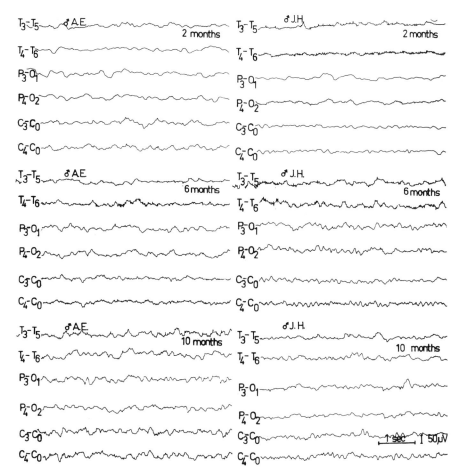

FIG. 17. EEGs from two children at three ages. To the left "slow," to the right "fast" type of record.

type of EEG and steeply rising regression lines characterize the "fast" type of EEG in the second child.

DISCUSSION

The 60-sec epoch length in spectral analysis is the same as that used in the broadband analysis, and the sections chosen visually for analysis are identical in both analyses. This epoch length was chosen partly for practical rea-

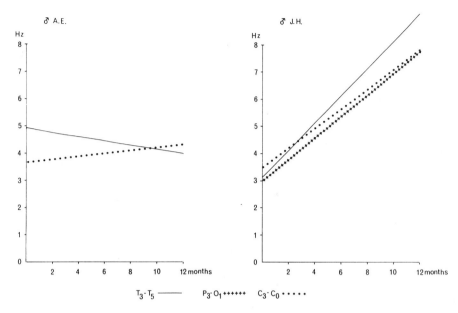

FIG. 18. Regression lines of development of peak frequency in the same infants as in Fig. 17. To the left: slight upward or even downward course of regression lines corresponding to the "slow" type of record (in the parieto-occipital lead no regression line due to lack of points). To the right: steeply rising regression lines of the "fast" type of EEG.

recordings in broadband analysis through the analysis of two 60-sec periods in the same trace. The standard error of a single determination was approximately 10% for the delta and theta bands. Corbin and Bickford (1955) made analyses of epoch lengths varying from 10 to 80 sec and found great constancy in the pattern from one and the same cortical region ("when environmental and subjective variables are reduced to a minimum"). Stability was not less in young groups than in older groups. An analysis time of 3×10 sec was decided upon. Dumermuth, who has performed spectral analysis via FFT in children and young adults (1968, 1969) with five to six 50-sec epochs, also found great agreement among different epochs. Therefore, a 60-sec period of analysis is likely to provide a reliable estimate of the frequency spectrum in awake infants.

It is of interest to compare the variability found among spectra for a certain age and lead with those derived theoretically in the Appendix. In the case of a signal of normal distribution, the spectral estimator was found to be distributed as a chi-squared variable with 98 degrees of freedom. From this a coefficient of variation of $\sqrt{2/98} = 0.14$ is derived, *i.e.*, considerably less than that found empirically when individuals were compared. This is in (qualitative) agreement with the inter-individual variations to be expected.

In all frequency analysis, the quality of the original EEG records is naturally of fundamental importance. The record should be free from artifacts, and the degree of wakefulness should be defined carefully by parameters other than EEG patterns. These requirements are especially difficult to satisfy in respect to infants, who are almost always in motion. Movement artifacts are therefore almost unavoidable. Awake recordings with closed eyes, customary in adults and older children, are impossible in this age group, in which open eyes are the only practically usable, objective criterion of alertness. Within the limits of this definition, there may be variation from maximal alertness to mild drowsiness. Moreover, when the eyes are open, blocking of dominant activity caused by visual or attention factors may occur, thereby changing the frequency spectrum. According to Corbin and Bickford (1955), visual blocking is relatively modest before the second year of life, even if inter-individual variations are great, and Grey Walter (1953) has reported that not until 3 or 4 years of age is an unmistakable effect on the alpha-rhythm by visual stimulation found. On the other hand, Lindsley (1938) felt that "the alpha rhythm" was blocked by visual or other stimuli even in children a few months old. A similar view was subsequently advanced by many authors, including Dreyfus-Brisac and Blanc (1956) and Dreyfus-Brisac, Samson, Blanc, and Monod (1958) who, however, like Corbin and Bickford, found that the effect of eye opening is variable at this age. The visual blocking effect was not especially studied in our investigation, but we also noted that this effect can vary considerably among children in the same age group (Fig. 19), a circumstance which may contribute to the inter-individual variation in the spectral curves. Differences in the degree of blocking by attention, visual or other stimuli may also be responsible for abrupt intra-individual changes in peak height and peak frequency from one age to another, as e.g., the peak frequencies illustrated in Fig. 11C. When the dot diagram for peak frequency (Fig. 10) is studied, it is striking to note, at least with respect to the parieto-occipital and central regions, that the dots, from about the age of 6 months, are distributed in two groups: a larger, high-frequency, rather tightly bunched group, and a smaller group with values far below the regression line with almost no values in between. This distribution may possibly be due to the fact that peaks in the former group represent true dominant activity, whereas values in the low-frequency group may represent the frequency that dominates after blocking of the dominant activity. Clinically nondiscernible differences in degree of wakefulness may also have contributed to the large variations in peak frequency.

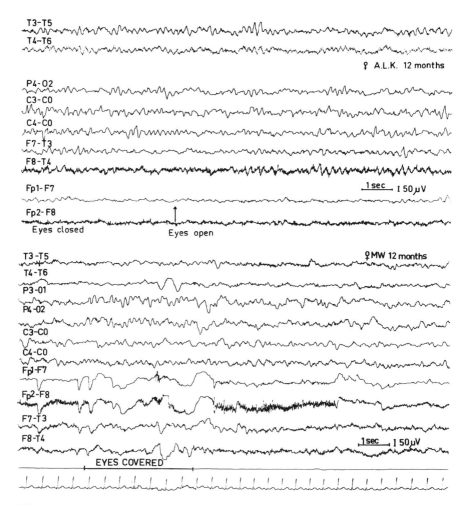

FIG. 19. Effect of eye opening in two infants of the same age. *Upper record:* rhythmic activity ceases on eye opening but returns after a few seconds. *Lower record:* rhythmic activity present when the baby's eyes are covered, practically absent with eyes open.

evaluation and frequency analysis, in that low-frequency activity, mainly in the delta region, dominates. The relative share of low-frequency activity declined successively, which is characteristic of EEG development throughout childhood. The spread in the mean spectrum was relatively great and at a maximum in the peak region. The large standard deviation in this region reflects large inter-individual differences in peak frequency and peak height, as the special studies of frequency peaks disclosed. Mizuno, Yamauchi,

Watanabe, Komatsushiro, Takagi, Iinuma and Arakawa (1970) obtained no distinct frequency peaks at all in mean spectra from 3-, 6- and 12-month-old children in the right occipital region, probably because of a combination of great variability among individuals and small sample sizes. In Corbin and Bickford's mean compounded frequency spectra from the parieto-occipital region, there was only a hint of a 5–6 Hz hump at the age of 1 year.

The central region differed considerably from the other two regions analyzed, which in themselves displayed great similarities in the pattern of development. An earlier frequency peak, a higher frequency of this peak and a greater peak height occurred centrally, the latter variable reflecting amplitude and constancy of the dominant rhythm. The central dominant rhythm in visual evaluation as well often appeared in long continuous sequences. This apparently more advanced development of the EEG in the central region probably corresponds to the greater morphological differentiation in the motor cortex region as compared to other cortical regions, as described by Conel (1939–1955) for newborns and older infants.

With respect to possible sex differences, a tendency to a higher peak frequency is seen in girls than in boys. This finding is of interest in view of the higher frequency for the alpha rhythm in girls than in boys, that Lindsley found visually as early as 1938, subsequently confirmed by Henry (1944) and recently by Petersén and Eeg-Olofsson (1970–1971) in a study of normal children from 1–15 years. With a larger sample of normal infants, it might be possible to demonstrate that a sex differentiation of the EEG begins as early as the first year of life.

In comparisons between visual and spectral analysis peak frequency, the spread was greater with automatic determination. Mean values agreed rather well in the two methods, but there could be great discrepancy in individual cases. Automatic spectral analysis, which is completely objective, indicates the frequency of greatest intensity during the period covered by the analysis. Visual evaluation is often based on a longer period of recording than spectral analysis, since the eye can also make use of very brief sections of EEG in quietness between movement artifacts. Therefore, visual evaluation can occasionally be more efficient than automatic evaluation. This may explain why a "dominant activity" was often found visually, especially in the younger age groups, when there were no peak frequencies in the spectra. As previously mentioned, there was occasionally more than a single peak. In such cases the secondary peak rather than the highest peak sometimes corresponded to visual dominant activity. As pointed out by Pechstein (1970a), visual evaluation primarily means a search for rhythms and pat-

even with respect to the frequency of the background activity. Extreme values may be unconsciously avoided in favor of "normal" frequencies, which would explain the smaller spreads in visual evaluation. Peak frequency in spectral analysis and dominant activity in visual evaluation are, thus, two somewhat different concepts: in the former case an objectively evaluated true dominant frequency, in the latter case a subjectively determined rhythm which, although perhaps only occurring to a limited extent, resembles a "dominant activity."

To summarize, one could say that spectral analysis via FFT of the EEG from normal infants has provided a detailed picture of frequency spectrum development, generally and individually. Interest has primarily centered on the development of the dominant frequency, for which broadband analysis can provide no information. Many who have studied the EEG of normal infants have emphasized its great variability. This view, with respect to the awake EEG, has been confirmed and perhaps even reinforced by spectral analysis, providing an objective measure of the variability. The great breadth of inter- and intra-individual variation restricts the usefulness of spectral analysis in clinical diagnosis for this age group. Another factor of importance to the clinical use of the method on infant materials is the difficulty in obtaining technically satisfactory awake recordings. Despite all this, we feel that the method may be useful in selected cases in this age group, *e.g.*, in order to follow the course of a disorder or the effect of treatment. With appropriate modifications, the FFT method should be applicable to the EEG of older children and adults to a greater extent. For the time being, however, spectral analysis cannot replace the conventional evaluation of the EEG but can supplement it.

SUMMARY

The EEG development of a selected group of 29 healthy infants has been studied from birth to 1 year of age with examinations at 2-month intervals which included EEG recording, and neurological state and developmental tests. Visual evaluation and broadband frequency analysis of the waking records had been performed earlier. The waking EEGs of 20 infants from the same material have now been subjected to a spectral analysis via Fast Fourier Transform (FFT). From three cortical regions in each hemisphere, 60-sec artifact-free segments were used for spectral analysis. After analog-to-digital conversion, the power spectrum was calculated via FFT, using a spectral window of 0.4 Hz half-power width. After factorization of each spectrum into a regression line and a remaining fluctuating component, peaks were extracted from the latter. Spectra were studied especially regarding occurrence of spectral peaks, and frequency and height of these peaks. In addition, the slope and mean intensity of the spectral curves were calculated.

Presence of peaks, peak frequency and peak height generally increased with age, whereas the slope of the spectral curves became less negative, the latter variable reflecting an increase of faster and a decrease of slower components. Inter- and intraindividual variations were great, and there were differences between the three cortical regions studied in each hemisphere. Differences between homologous areas, however, were generally small. The results have been compared, where possible, with the visual evaluation and the broadband analysis of the same records. The agreement between the three methods was good, as a rule, but in individual cases there were discrepancies between the visual and FFT evaluations.

Spectral analysis via FFT gives an objective numerical expression of EEG development. A disadvantage of automatic analysis is the demand for technically good EEG recordings, a demand which is specially hard to fulfill in small infants. Visual evaluation, owing to the filtering capacity of the eye, can make use also of technically imperfect parts of a record. As automatic analysis yields information of a character partly different from that furnished by visual analysis, the two methods are concluded to be mutually supplementary.

APPENDIX. THE SPECTRAL ESTIMATOR

by Jan Persson

1. Derivation

The method of using a modified, average periodogram [formulas (A-1)–(A-7), (A-13)], was proposed by Welch (1967).

Let the EEG, $x(t)$, be sampled with an interval of Δt, thus constituting a discrete time series $X(j)$. By sectioning the record into L segments of length T, with an overlap of 50%, L series $X_l(j)$ are obtained, as follows:

$$X_l(j) = X\left[j + (l-1)\frac{N}{2}\right], \tag{A-1}$$

where $N = T/\Delta t$, and $j = 0, 1, \ldots, N-1; l = 1, 2, \ldots, L$.

$$A_l(k) = \frac{1}{N} \sum_{j=0}^{N-1} X_l(j)W(j)W_N^{-jk}, \; l = 1, 2, \ldots, L, \tag{A-2}$$

where $W_N = e^{i2\pi/N}$, the segment periodogram

$$I_l(k) = \frac{T}{U} |A_l(k)|^2, \; k = 0, 1, \ldots, N/2, \tag{A-3}$$

where $U = \frac{1}{N} \sum_{j=0}^{N-1} W^2(j)$, and the average periodogram

$$I(k) = \frac{1}{L} \sum_{l=1}^{L} I_l(k), \; k = 0, 1, \ldots, N/2. \tag{A-4}$$

It is well known (Welch, 1967) that

$$E[I(k)] = \int_0^F p(f)q_l(k\Delta f - f)df, \tag{A-5}$$

where $q_l(f)$, the spectral window corresponding to the data window $W(j)$, has the properties

$$q_l(f) = \frac{1}{FUN} \left| \sum_{j=0}^{N-1} W(j)e^{-i2\pi jf/F} \right|^2 \tag{A-6}$$

and

$$\int_0^F q_l(f)df = 1. \tag{A-7}$$

The functions $X_l(j)$ and $W(j)$ are shown in Fig. 4.

The final spectral estimator $\hat{P}(k)$ is a sum of $(2R + 1)$ periodogram values, weighted by the sequence $Q(r), r = -R, -R + 1, \ldots, R$, for which $\sum_{-R}^{R} Q(r) = 1$:

$$\hat{P}(k) = \sum_{r=-R}^{R} Q(r)I(k + r), \; R \leq k \leq \frac{N}{2} - R. \tag{A-8}$$

This is more conveniently expressed if the set of weights $Q(r)$ is periodically continued with period N:

$$\hat{P}(k) = \sum_{m=0}^{N-1} I(m)Q(k - m), \; R \leq k \leq \frac{N}{2} - R, \tag{A-9}$$

where $\sum_{m=0}^{N-1} Q(m) = 1$.

Now let $\Delta f = 1/T$, $F = N \cdot \Delta f$, and suppose that the true EEG spectrum,

$p(f)$, vanishes above $f = F/2$. Then, using the periodicity of q_I and Q, it follows that:

$$E[\hat{P}(k)] = E\left[\sum_{m=0}^{N-1} I(m)Q(k-m)\right] =$$

$$= \sum_{m=0}^{N-1} \int_0^F p(f)q_I(m\Delta f - f)df Q(k-m) =$$

$$= \int_0^F p(f) \sum_{m=0}^{N-1} q_I[(k-m)\Delta f - f] \, Q(m)df =$$

$$= \int_0^F p(f)q_P(k\Delta f - f)df, \tag{A-10}$$

where

$$q_P(f) = \sum_{m=0}^{N-1} q_I(f - m\Delta f)Q(m). \tag{A-11}$$

It follows immediately that

$$\int_0^F q_P(f)df = 1. \tag{A-12}$$

These results have also been derived by Cooley, Lewis and Welch (1967, 1970).

Thus, the expected value of $\hat{P}(k)$ is the convolution between the true spectrum and a spectral window $q_P(f)$ of unit area. This means that, if the side lobes of the spectral window are negligible and the power spectrum is flat within the main lobe, then $\hat{P}(k)$ is an approximately unbiased estimator of the spectral density.

The $(1 - t^2)$-shaped data window applied, $W(j)$, implies (Welch, 1967) that $q_I(f) \approx q(f)$ in the range $-F/2 \leqslant f \leqslant F/2$, where

$$q(f) = \frac{15}{8T} \left\{ \frac{2T}{(\pi f T)^2} \left[\frac{\sin(\pi f T)}{\pi f T} - \cos(\pi f T) \right] \right\}^2. \tag{A-13}$$

The segment length used is $T = 10 \, s$, and the set of weights Q is

$$Q(0) = 0.248,$$
$$Q(1) = Q(-1) = 0.210,$$
$$Q(2) = Q(-2) = 0.124$$

The spectral window $q_P(f)$, the envelope of which is shown in Fig. 5, has a 3-dB bandwidth B_q of about $4.0/T = 0.4$ Hz.

2. Variability

Suppose that the EEG signal is white, stationary, Gaussian and of zero mean. Then the variance of $\hat{P}(k)$ is

$$\text{Var}[\hat{P}(k)] = E[\hat{P}^2(k)] - E^2[\hat{P}(k)], \tag{A-15}$$

where

$$E[\hat{P}(k)] = E[I(k)] \cdot \sum_{r=-R}^{R} Q(r), \tag{A-16}$$

and

$$E[\hat{P}^2(k)] = E\left[\sum_{r, s=-R}^{R} I(k-r)I(k-s)Q(r)Q(s)\right]. \tag{A-17}$$

If $I(k)$ and $I(l)$ are considered uncorrelated for $k \neq l$ (Jenkins and Watts, 1968), it follows that

$$E[\hat{P}^2(k)] = \text{Var}\ [I] \sum_{r=-R}^{R} Q^2(r) + E^2[I]. \tag{A-18}$$

Now introduce the normalized standard errors of $\hat{P}$, $\epsilon_{\hat{P}} = \sqrt{\text{Var}\ [\hat{P}]}/E[\hat{P}]$, and of I, $\epsilon_I = \sqrt{\text{Var}[I]}/E[I]$, and note that $\Sigma Q(r) = 1$. Then we have

$$\epsilon_{\hat{P}} = \epsilon_I \sqrt{\sum_{r=-R}^{R} Q^2(r)}. \tag{A-19}$$

The number of overlapping segments used is $L = 11$. As demonstrated by Welch (1967), we then have $\epsilon_I = \frac{1}{3}$, which, inserted in (A-19) together with the set of weights $Q(r)$, yields

$$\epsilon_{\hat{P}} \approx 0.143. \tag{A-20}$$

Thus the equivalent number ν of degrees of freedom of $\hat{P}$ is

$$\nu = 2/\epsilon_{\hat{P}}^2 = 98. \tag{A-21}$$

From the chi-squared distribution with 98 degrees of freedom, the one-sided 99% confidence limit for the spectrum is derived, with the following result:

$$\text{Prob}[\hat{P}(k)/p(k\Delta f) > 1.3 dB] = 1\%. \tag{A-22}$$

Thus, in a set of independent spectral estimates of a white, stationary, Gaussian signal, 1% will exceed a level of 1.3dB above the true spectral density.

ACKNOWLEDGMENT

This investigation was supported by a grant from the Swedish Medical Research Council.

REFERENCES

Arakawa, T., Mizuno, T., Chiba, F., Sakai, K., Watanabe, S., and Tamura, T. (1968): Frequency analysis of electroencephalograms and latency of photically induced average evoked responses in children with ariboflavinosis. *Tohoku Journal of Experimental Medicine*, 94:327–335.

Bartoshuk, A. K. (1964): Human neonatal EEG: Frequency analysis of awake and asleep samples from four areas. *Psychonomic Science*, 1:281–282.

Bartoshuk, A. K., and Tennant, J. M. (1964): Human neonatal EEG correlates of sleep-wakefulness and neural maturation. *Journal of Psychiatric Research*, 2:73–83.

Bergland, G. (1969): A radix-eight fast Fourier transform subroutine for real-valued series. *Institute of Electrical and Electronics Engineers Transactions on Audio Electroacoustics*, AU–17:138–144.

Bernhard, C. G., and Skoglund, C. R. (1939): On the alpha frequency of human brain potentials as a function of age. *Skandinavisches Archiv für Physiologie*, 82:178–184.

Conel, J. L. (1939–1955): *The Postnatal Development of the Human Cerebral Cortex*. Harvard University Press, Cambridge, Mass.

Cooley, J. W., Lewis, P. A. W., and Welch, P. D. (Feb. 1967): The fast Fourier transform and its applications. *IBM Research Report RC 1743*, 157 pp.

Cooley, J. W., Lewis, P. A. W., and Welch, P. D. (1970): The application of the fast Fourier transform algorithm to the estimation of spectra and cross-spectra. *Journal of Sound Vibration*, 12:339–352.

Cooley, J. W., and Tukey, J. W. (1965): An algorithm for the machine calculation of complex Fourier series. *Mathematics of Computation*, 19:297–301.

Corbin, H. P. F., and Bickford, R. G. (1955): Studies of the electroencephalogram of normal children: comparison of visual and automatic frequency analyses. *Electroencephalography and Clinical Neurophysiology*, 7:15–28.

Dreyfus-Brisac, C., and Blanc, C. (1956): Aspects électroencéphalographiques de la maturation cérébrale pendant la première année de la vie. *Electroencephalography and Clinical Neurophysiology*, Suppl. 6:432–440.

Dreyfus-Brisac, C., Samson, D., Blanc, C., and Monod, N. (1958): L'électroencéphalogramme de l'enfant normal de moins de 3 ans. Aspect fonctionel bioélectrique de la maturation nerveuse. *Études Néo-Natales*, VII, 4:143–175.

Drohocki, Z., and Duflo, G. (1958): L'électrochronogramme du cerveau chez l'enfant normal et ses modifications sous l'influence de l'hyperpnée. *Journal de Physiologie (Paris)*, 50:251–255.

Dumermuth, G. (1968): Variance spectra of electroencephalograms in twins. A contribution to the problem of quantification of EEG background activity in childhood. In: *Clinical Electroencephalography of Children*, edited by P. Kellaway and I. Petersén. Almqvist & Wiksell,

Dumermuth, G. (1971): Electronic data processing in pediatric EEG research. *Neuropädiatrie*, 2:349–374.

Dumermuth, G. Numerical spectral analysis of the electroencephalogram. In: *International Handbook of Electroencephalography and Clinical Neurophysiology*, edited by A. Rémond. Elsevier Publishing Co., Amsterdam (*in press*).

Fujimori, B., Yokota, T., Ishibashi, Y., and Takel, T. (1958): Analysis of the electroencephalogram of children by histogram method. *Electroencephalography and Clinical Neurophysiology*, 10:241–242.

Gabersek, V., and Scherrer, J. (1966): Etude électrophysiologique du sommeil de l'enfant. *Revue de Neuropsychiatrie Infantile*, 14:121–138.

Gibbs, F. A., and Knott, J. R. (1949): Growth of the electrical activity of the cortex. *Electroencephalography and Clinical Neurophysiology*, 1:223–229.

Hagne, I. (1968): Development of the waking EEG in normal infants during the first year of life. In: *Clinical Electroencephalography of Children*, edited by P. Kellaway and I. Petersén. Almqvist & Wiksell, Stockholm, pp. 97–118.

Hashimoto, Y., and Hamava, K. (1963): A frequency analysis of electroencephalograms of healthy children and youths. *Kobe Journal of Medical Science*, 9:89–92.

Henry, C. E. (1944): Electroencephalograms of normal children. Society for Research in Child Development, Washington, IX, No. 3.

Jenkins, G. M., and Watts, D. G. (1968): *Spectral Analysis and Its Applications*. Holden-Day, San Francisco.

Knott, J. R., and Gibbs, F. A. (1939): A Fourier transform of the EEG from one to eighteen years. *Psychological Bulletin*, 36:512–513.

Lairy, G. C., Rémond, A., Rieger, H., and Lesèvre, N. (1969): The alpha average. III. Clinical application in children. *Electroencephalography and Clinical Neurophysiology*, 26:453–467.

Lindsley, D. B. (1938): Electrical potentials of the brain in children and adults. *Journal of General Psychology*, 19:285–306.

Lindsley, D. B. (1939): A longitudinal study of the occipital alpha rhythm in normal children: frequency and amplitude standards. *Journal of Genetic Psychology*, 55:197–213.

Matoušek, M., and Petersén, I. Frequency analysis of the EEG in normal children and adolescents. (*this volume*.)

Mizuno, T., Yamauchi, N., Watanabe, A., Komatsushiro, M., Takagi, T., Iinuma, K., and Arakawa, T. (1970): Maturation patterns of EEG basic waves of healthy infants under twelve months of age. *Tohoku Journal of Experimental Medicine*, 102:91–98.

Nolte, R., Schulte, F. J., Michaelis, R., and Juergens, U. (1968): Power spectral analysis of the electroencephalogram of newborn twins in active and quiet sleep. In: *Clinical Electroencephalography of Children*, edited by P. Kellaway and I. Petersén. Almqvist & Wiksell, Stockholm, pp. 89–96.

Nolte, R., Schulte, F. J., Michaelis, R., Weisse, U., and Gruson, R. (1969): Bioelectric brain maturation in small-for-dates infants. *Developmental Medicine and Child Neurology*, 11:83–93.

Parmelee, A. H., Akiyama, Y., Schultz, M. A., Wenner, W. H., and Schulte, F. J. (1969): Analysis of the electroencephalogram of sleeping infants. *Activitas Nervosa Superior*, 11-2:111–115.

Pechstein, J. (1970*a*): Entwicklung der Grundaktivität im frühkindlichen EEG. Der TAM-Wert als brauchbare Masszahl der Dominanz im Wach-EEG der ersten beiden Lebensjahre. *Fortschritte der Medizin*, 88:1170–1176.

Pechstein, J. (1970*b*): Konstanz des Theta-Alpha-Medianwertes (TAM-Wertes) im kindlichen EEG-Frequenzspektrum bei geöffneten und geschlossenen Augen. EEG-EMG, 1:107–110.

Pechstein, J., and Dolansky, J. (1970): Zur Methodik der visuellen Frequenzanalyse des Wach-EEG im frühen Kindesalter. EEG-EMG, 1:35–39.

Persson, J. (1971): A computerized spectral analysis of electroencephalograms from normal children during the first year of life. Thesis, Departments of Electrical Measurements and Applied Electronics, Chalmers University of Technology, and Clinical Neurophysiology, Sahlgren Hospital, Göteborg.

Petersén, I., and Eeg-Olofsson, O. (1971): The development of the electroencephalogram in normal children from the age of 1 through 15 years. Non-paroxysmal activity. *Neuropädiatrie*, 2:247–304.

Prechtl, H. F. (1968): Polygraphic studies of the full-term newborn. II. Computer analysis of recorded data. *Clinics in Developmental Medicine*, 27:22–40.

Prechtl, H. F., Weinmann, H., and Akiyama, Y. (1969): Organization of physiological parameters in normal and neurologically abnormal infants. *Neuropädiatrie*, 1:101–129.

Rémond, A., Lesèvre, N., Joseph, J. P., Rieger, H., and Lairy, G. C. (1969): The alpha average. I. Methodology and description. *Electroencephalography and Clinical Neurophysiology*, 26:245–265.

Scheffner, D. (1968): Eine einfache Methode zur quantitativen Bestimmung langsamer Frequenzen im EEG von Kindern. *Archiv für Kinderheilk*, 177:41–48.

Schulte, F. J., Hinze, G., and Schrempf, G. (1971): Maternal toxemia, fetal malnutrition and bioelectric brain activity of the newborn. *Neuropädiatrie*, 2:439–460.

Walter, W. G. (1950): Normal rhythms—their development, distribution and significance. In: *Electroencephalography*, edited by D. Hill and G. Parr. Macdonald, London, pp. 203–227.

Walter, W. G. (1953): *The Living Brain*. Gerald Duckworth & Co., Ltd., London, pp. 137–140.

Welch, P. D. (1967): The use of fast Fourier transform for the estimation of power spectra: A method based on time averaging over short, modified periodograms. *Institute of Electrical and Electronics Engineers Transactions on Audio Electroacoustics*, AU–15:70–73.

DISCUSSION

In discussing this paper, Kellaway made two points. (1) Some of the discrepancies between visual and FFT evaluations may have been at least partly due to the electroencephalographer "seeing what he expected to see" in the EEGs from a particular age group, although other explanations may apply in particular situations, and some of these had been mentioned in the report. (2) In establishing normal criteria for children's EEGs, it will be necessary to establish certain montages in order to be able to compare data from different institutions. For example, it is probably important that the recording technique include a derivation from the central region, since an ontogenetically interesting activity is often seen in that region. This activity consists of an 8/sec rhythm which is present in a proportion of newborn infants and which seems to disappear for a while and then reappear later on.

Automation of Clinical Electroencephalography.
Edited by P. Kellaway and I. Petersén.
Raven Press, New York © 1973.

EEG Spectral Analysis by Means of Fast Fourier Transform

G. Dumermuth and E. Keller

Department of Electroencephalography, Children's Hospital, University of Zurich, Zurich, Switzerland

Through the pioneering work of D. O. Walter and his co-workers (e.g., Walter, 1963; Walter and Adey, 1965; Walter and Adey, 1966; Walter, Kado, Rhodes, and Adey, 1967; Adey, Kado, and Walter, 1967), digital spectral analysis was introduced into electroencephalography as a most promising quantification and analysis technique. However, until recently digital spectral analysis could be performed only where large computing facilities together with a considerable amount of computer time were available.

The most important advance to change this situation was made in 1965, when a fast computational procedure was rediscovered which permitted the calculation of Fourier coefficients of discrete periodic functions in an economical way (Cooley and Tukey, 1965). This algorithm quickly became famous under the name Fast Fourier Transform (FFT). Furthermore, the modern computer industry offers small and fast laboratory computer systems for reasonable prices. Therefore, spectral analysis may be performed in the EEG laboratory, which makes this method even more attractive today.

Spectral analysis treats the amplitude of the EEG as a random variable. The *power spectrum* (autospectrum, variance spectrum)

$$S(\omega) = E[Z(\omega)Z^*(\omega)]$$

(where Z represents the Fourier transform of the signal, $*$ its complex con-

145

jugate, and $E[\ ]$ the expected value of the quantity within the brackets when measured over an infinite period of time) gives an estimate of the mean square value or average intensity of the EEG as a function of frequency. It displays the decomposition of the total variability or variance into contributions from the individual frequency bands.

The *cross-spectrum*

$$S_{xy}(\omega) = E[Z_x(\omega)Z_y^*(\omega)]$$

provides information about statistical interrelationships (covariance) between two simultaneous EEG records (X and Y) in the frequency domain. It allows the computation of two important quantities, *i.e.*, the coherence spectrum

$$C_{xy}(\omega) = \frac{|S_{xy}(\omega)|^2}{S_x(\omega)S_y(\omega)}$$

and the phase spectrum $\varphi_{xy}(\omega) = \arg S_{xy}(\omega)$.

The coherence is a measure of the correlation between two EEG records for each frequency band, and the phase spectrum displays the average phase difference between the correlated (phase-locked) frequency components.

Spectral analysis provides in principle the same information as correlation analysis as the results form a Fourier transform pair (Fig. 1). However, the spectral representation has important statistical advantages over correlation analysis; it also corresponds more to the conventional description of the background activity of the EEG in terms of relative frequency content.

Spectral analysis is a powerful analytical tool with well-behaving statistical properties as long as certain assumptions about the nature of the data (especially normal distribution of the amplitudes and stationariness) are not grossly violated. If the data are stationary, i.e., do not change their statistical properties with time, spectral estimates do not depend upon the assumption of a normal amplitude distribution (Blackman and Tukey, 1958). In the non-Gaussian case, however, they will reflect only part of the information. It is important to note this restriction, as our recent studies have shown that actual EEG data are rarely Gaussian. Also the assumption of stationariness is valid only for relatively short epochs of EEG data (e.g., waking activity at rest; Dumermuth, 1968, 1969), whereas in sleep or during behavioral or performance tests the EEG is certainly not stationary. However, despite objections from theorists of time series analysis, spectral analysis of non-stationary EEGs of, for example, sleep activity may provide very useful information (Adey, Kado and Walter, 1967; Walter, Kado, Rhodes, and Adey, 1967; Dumermuth, Huber, Keiner and Gasser, 1970; Dumermuth, 1970; Dumermuth, Walz, Scollo-Lavizzarri and Kleiner, 1972; Fig. 8).

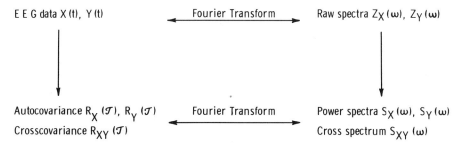

FIG. 1. Mathematical relationships between EEG data, covariance functions and spectra. The raw spectra $Z(\omega)$ are complex quantities composed of sine and cosine components or in polar representation, of amplitude and phase.

Computational Procedures

To calculate spectral estimates, different approaches are possible: *digital bandpass filtering* (Ormsby, 1961); *Fourier transform of correlograms* (indirect method; Blackman and Tukey, 1958); *direct Fourier transform* (direct method; for references see Dumermuth and Flühler, 1967).

Like almost everybody before 1965, we started our own work by using the indirect method. However, we soon realized that a broader application of spectral analysis was out of the question because of the large amount of computer time consumed by the calculation of the mean lagged products. During this time, D. O. Walter had already begun to use digital bandpass filtering (Walter and Adey, 1966). The introduction of the FFT in 1965 meant for us a drastic change from an otherwise almost hopeless situation; it then became possible to use the direct method with a considerable saving of computer time. After we had implemented the FFT into a new program, the computer time needed to perform the same analysis was reduced by a factor of approximately 50 (Dumermuth and Flühler, 1967; Kleiner, Flühler, Huber and Dumermuth, 1970).

Fast Fourier Transform (FFT)

In 1965 Cooley and Tukey published a first version of a fast algorithm for the calculation of the Fourier coefficients of discrete periodic functions. It is evident that using classical formulas to calculate the Fourier coefficients in a straightforward way is not economical because a large part of the sums and products are calculated more than once. The FFT avoids this computational redundancy. For $N = 2^m$, only about $2N \log_2 N$ arithmetic operations are required instead of N^2 operations in the classical procedure.

For a detailed outline of the FFT algorithm we refer to the publications of Gentleman and Sande (1966), Cochran, Cooley, Favin, Helms, Kaenel, Lang, Maling, Nelson, Rader and Welch (1967), Rothman (1968) and Bergland (1969). Fortunately, many computer companies include a binary coded subroutine of the FFT in their software package. Thus, the FFT may be implemented without further programming effort, which was not possible until approximately 5 years ago.

Windows: Leakage and Spectral Stability

Spectral quantities are statistical descriptors of the data. As in ordinary statistics, only estimates from finite samples are possible. However, an EEG record of length T may be thought of as complemented by zeroes outside the observation epoch, T. This is equivalent to multiplication of the infinite time series $X(t)$ with a rectangular gate function $G(t)$ of amplitude 1 between $-T/2 \leq 0 \leq T/2$ and zero outside. The gate function $G(t)$ may be regarded as a time window through which the observer looks at $X(t)$. Multiplication of $X(t)$ with the gate function $G(t)$ corresponds to convolution of the Fourier transform of $X(t)$ with the Fourier transform of $G(t)$, i.e., to smoothing of the spectrum of $X(t)$ with the spectrum of $G(t)$. The latter is called a spectral window $W(\omega)$ and has the well-known form of the sampling function $\sin X/X$ (Fig. 2).

A most annoying property of the spectral window function $W(\omega)$ consists in the slow decay of its side lobes. The consequence is a considerable overlapping of adjacent frequency bands which introduces mutual correlation between the different Fourier coefficients and the spectral quantities derived from these. This disturbing side effect is called leakage. To reduce leakage, window modifications are necessary, which may be performed either in the frequency or in the time domain. A popular procedure consists in "Hanning" (Blackman and Tukey, 1958), i.e., smoothing the sine and cosine series by the weights $-\frac{1}{4}$, $\frac{1}{2}$, $-\frac{1}{4}$ (for data defined between 0 and T when using the FFT). Instead of smoothing the Fourier coefficients, we may also modify the data window by "tapering" both ends. Hanning in the time domain, e.g., is accomplished by replacing the rectangular window by a cosine bell-shaped window function $\frac{1}{2}\left(1 - \cos 2\pi \frac{t}{T}\right)$. Hanning leads to a much faster decay of the side lobes and reduces leakage considerably. As Bingham, Godfrey and Tukey (1967) point out, any such correction for leakage must be done directly on the sine and cosine coefficients and not on the spectral quantitites derived from these. This point has to be emphasized because most discussions on spectral windows were written at a time when spectral analysis was performed by the indirect method.

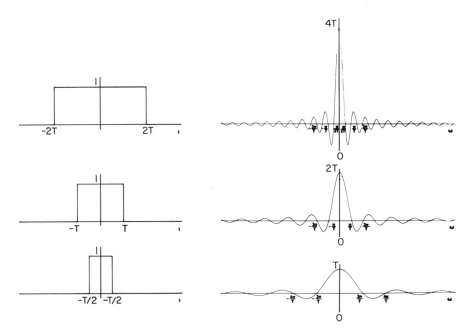

FIG. 2. Time and spectral windows. A: time windows $G(t)$ of variable length, B: their corresponding spectral window $W(\omega)$. Compression in the time domain is equivalent to expansion in the frequency domain.

Raw and Smoothed Periodograms

Combining the squares of the sine and cosine coefficients gives the famous periodogram. For a finite sample the corresponding spectral window has the form of $\sin^2 X/X^2$ (Figs. 3 and 4). The periodogram, however, is not a consistent estimate of the true spectrum, as its stability does not improve with increasing sample size. This is easily understood by the fact that increasing the number of data points only increases the number of spectral points without improving their individual significance.

To obtain consistent spectral estimates, *i.e.*, of higher stability, either smoothing over adjacent frequency bands or averaging a series of periodograms from several consecutive data sections has to be performed.

Some reasons for the smoothing procedure may also be explained as follows. Correlation transforms the rectangular time window into an isosceles triangle whose Fourier transform has the form of the squared sampling function ($\sin^2 X/X^2$), i.e., of the periodogram window (Fig. 4). In the actual case with data of finite length, the variance of the correlogram increases with increasing lag τ as less and less data contribute to the mean lagged products.

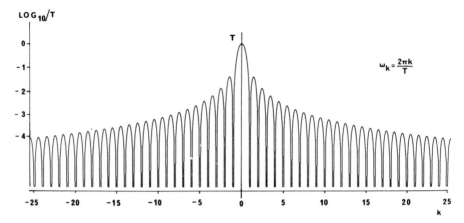

FIG. 3. Periodogram window. The window is plotted in a logarithmic scale. ω_k = frequency, $\Delta\omega = 2\pi/T$ and $\omega = 2\pi f$. The plot demonstrates the slow decay of the side lobes as ω_k recedes from ω_0, which explains possible effects from leakage between frequency bands.

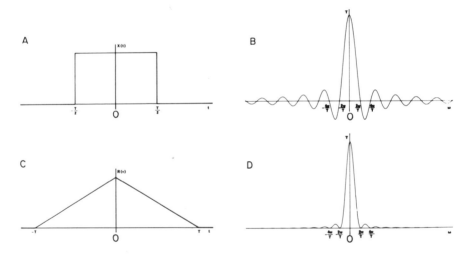

FIG. 4. Relationships between windows in the time and frequency domain. The rectangular data window function A forms a Fourier transform pair with the spectral window B. Autocorrelation of the data window gives a triangular window function C, which forms a Fourier transform pair with the periodogram window D.

Therefore, the correlation operation is terminated at a certain truncation point between $\tau = T/20$ and $\tau = T/5$ (Blackman and Tukey, 1958). Taking the Fourier transform of the truncated correlogram results in a broader spectral window. Truncating, therefore, has the same effect as smoothing,

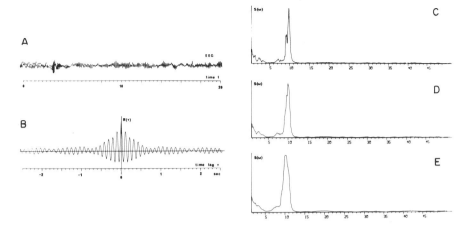

FIG. 5. Autocorrelogram and power spectrum. Normal adult control (female, 29 years) awake with eyes closed. A: Sample of the original record (P4 to right ear lobe). B: Correlogram (sampling rate 100/sec, total lag ± 256 points). C–D: Power spectra, smoothed over 7, 15, or 31 adjacent frequency bands, respectively. Spectral resolution therefore is 0.342 Hz for C, 0.732 Hz for D, and 1.515 Hz for E. The different spectral resolution corresponds to different truncation points in the correlogram at $\tau = 1.463$, 0.683, and 0.330 sec, respectively.

i.e., pooling weighted adjacent periodogram windows together into a correspondingly broader spectral window (Fig. 5).

Smoothing the periodogram increases the stability of the spectral estimates but reduces spectral resolution. In spectral analysis of actual EEG data, a compromise between stability and resolution has to be evaluated.

A different way to increase stability of the spectral estimates is sectioning the data and *averaging the periodograms* of consecutive pieces. Although the same basic spectral resolution and stability may be obtained for a record of a given length, the side lobes of the spectral window are much broader in this case and therefore leakage problems more serious. Welch (1967) proposes heavy tapering of the individual pieces and overlapping the sections to compensate for decreased stability. By overlapping the data pieces, the tapered parts of the data enter once more into the spectral estimation procedure. Although more calculations have to be performed, this approach may bring some advantages when a digital computer of restricted memory size (e.g., a 4k laboratory computer) is used.

Spectral Analysis in the EEG Laboratory

In preparing spectral analysis, one has to decide first whether to use large computer installations or to install small computer systems in the laboratory.

Large computer systems such as in university or hospital computing centers are generally not apt to handle large amount of EEG data because of the still-existing input/output difficulties in conventional computer systems. Furthermore, turn-around time is usually rather slow. Therefore, large conventional multi-user computer systems seem to be suitable only for small research projects where restricted amounts of EEG data may be processed in batch mode.

As already mentioned, the computer industry now provides small, general-purpose laboratory computer systems at reasonable prices. If properly programmed, these machines allow full-scale digital spectral analysis in the laboratory, either off-line or on-line. However, the programming effort for small machines must not be underestimated.

Small laboratory computer systems (e.g., the DEC PDP-12 with a memory cycle time of 1.6μsec, 12 bit words and 8k memory) may be expected to perform: (1) calculation of smoothed periodograms and their logarithm for two or three simultaneous EEG channels in real time, (2) calculation of logarithmic power spectra, coherence, phase and gain functions of two simultaneous EEG samples of 2048 points (i.e., 20 sec) each within less than 60 sec (excluding input and output), when using software floating-point arithmetic (Fig. 6), and (3) calculation of the same spectral quantities within 20 sec, when using a hardwired floating-point processor. This technique allows continuous cross-spectral analysis of two EEG channels in real time.

The development of hardwired FFT processors and similar accessories will further reduce computation time substantially. Therefore, it may be anticipated that digital spectral analysis will develop into a generally available laboratory procedure within the next few years.

Some Examples

In Figs. 6 to 8, examples of digitally calculated auto- and cross-spectra of EEG data are presented. Decisions regarding sampling frequency, sample length, spectral resolution and other parameters of analysis depend on the nature of the data to be analyzed and on the specific questions to be answered. A careful individual evaluation of these parameters before analysis is therefore to be recommended.

ACKNOWLEDGMENTS

The author thanks P. J. Huber and B. Kleiner (Department of Statistics, Swiss Federal Institute of Technology), and G. Scollo-Lavizzari (Department of Neurology, University of Basle) for their cooperation. The assist-

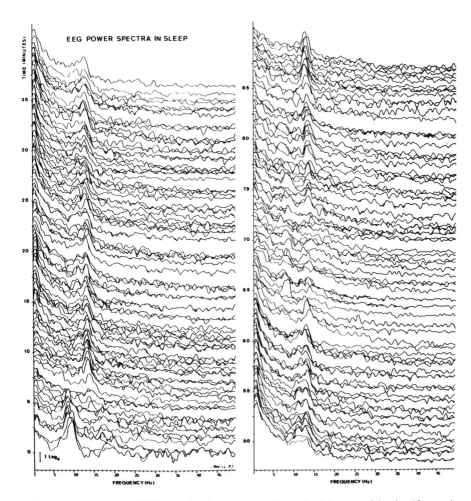

FIG. 6. Spectrogram of EEG activity during sleep. Normal adult control (male, 18 years). The plot shows the power spectra of the first cycle of an all-night sleep record from consecutive samples of 20 sec. Unipolar derivation from C4 to the right ear lobe. Time is in minutes; about 10 min is omitted between the first half (left) and the second half (right) of the spectrogram. The spectrogram displays the temporal behavior of the alpha-, sigma-, and delta-peaks and demonstrates the contrast between the well-organized time pattern of slow wave sleep and the disorganized pattern of REM sleep (middle part of the spectrogram at right). Spectral analysis was performed on a DEC PDP-12 laboratory computer system. Sample length is 20 sec (2,048 points), spectral resolution is 0.75 Hz.

ance of W. Walz, C. Brayshaw, W. and S. Adank and O. Brunner, Children's Hospital, is gratefully acknowledged.

This investigation was supported in part by the "Schweizerischer National-fonds zur Förderung der Wissenschaftlichen Forschung" (Nr. 3049 and

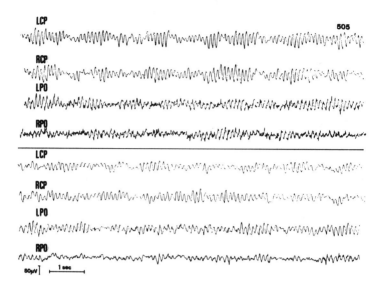

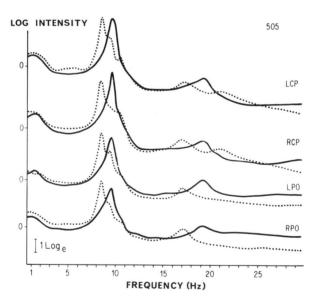

FIG. 7. EEG and Power Spectra in Twins (*cf.* Dumermuth, 1968, 1969). A: EEG and power spectra in a pair of nonidentical twins. Original record shows the background activity of both twins, simultaneously recorded with eyes closed (*upper part* subject A, *lower part* subject B. LCP = left centroparietal, RPO = right parieto-occipital region). The spectra (— subject A, – – – subject B) show the pronounced difference of the alpha peak frequency.

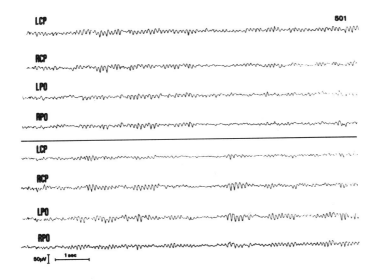

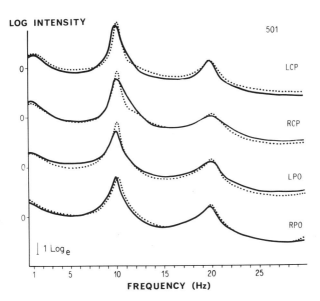

B: EEG and power spectra in a pair of identical twins. The power spectra confirm the identity of the statistical characteristics of the two records.

Spectral analysis was performed on the CDC 1604A–160A computer system of the Swiss Federal Institute of Technology in Zurich. Sample length is 40 sec (4,096 points), spectral resolution is 0.375 Hz.

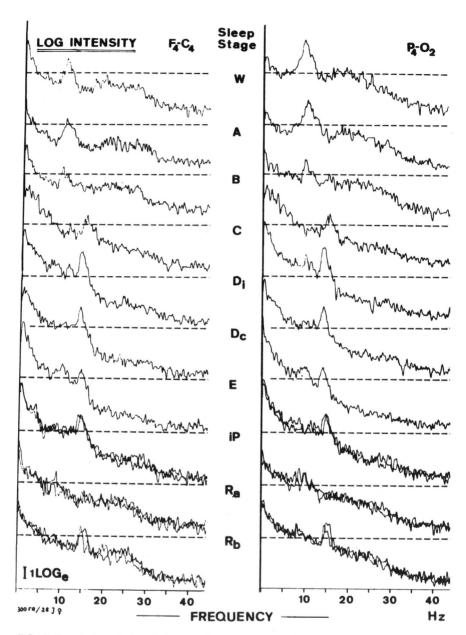

FIG. 8. Spectral analysis of sleep activity (*cf.* Dumermuth, Walz, Scollo-Lavizzari, and Kleiner, 1972). A: *Power spectra* of EEG samples taken from different sleep stages in a normal adult, female, age 28 years, during all-night sleep. Bipolar derivations F4–C4 and P4–O2. Sleep Stages: A, B, C, E according to Loomis, 1937; D_i, intermittent and D_c, continuous stage D; iP = intermediate phase (Schwartz, 1968); Ra = REM sleep with eye movements, Rb = REM sleep without eye movements but all other criteria for paradoxical sleep present. Logarithmic plot. Sample length is 40 sec (4,096 points), spectral resolution 0.375 Hz. The spectra display the different frequency content of the EEG activity for the various sleep stages and allow a quantitative comparison.

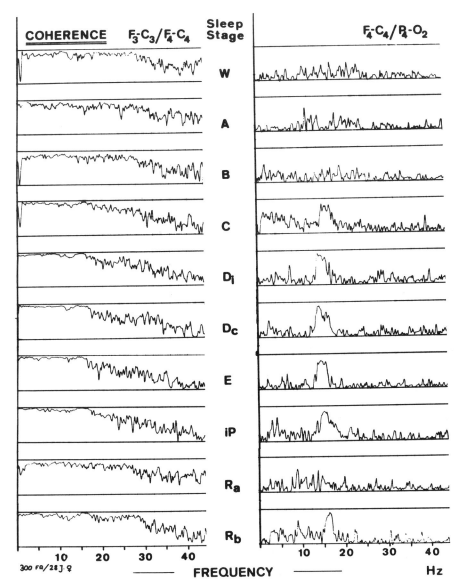

B: *Coherence spectra.* The left side shows coherence between the right and left fronto-central derivations which is high in the lower and middle part of the spectrum. The right side displays coherence between the fronto-central and the parieto-occipital derivations. Here, significant coherence is restricted to the frequency band of 13 to 16 Hz, corresponding to the sleep spindles, i.e., sigma activity. These findings imply a central pacemaker for sigma activity. Spectral analysis was performed as indicated in Fig. 7.

3.79.68), the "Emil-Barell-Stiftung der Fa. Hoffmann-La Roche zur Förderung der Medizinisch-Wissenschaftlichen Forschung" and the "Fritz Hoffmann-La Roche-Stiftung zur Förderung Wissenschaftlicher Arbeitsgemeinschaften in der Schweiz" (Nr. 111).

DISCUSSION

Dumermuth agreed with Walter, who commented that in situations where spectral analysis was used frequently for specific applications and where a certain fixed number of points was used in computing the spectrum, time was lost if standard FFT packages were used. It is possible to rewrite the FFT programs for a particular length at a saving of 20 to 30% in computation time.

Levy mentioned that he had heard experts state that parameter estimation methods of spectral analysis with long time series have some advantages in terms of computation speed over the FFT, and he asked Zetterberg if he could confirm this. Zetterberg replied that he had not made a direct comparison of the two methods, but a PDP-12 is currently being installed in his department, and he would hope to be able to give a definitive answer to the question in the near future. However, it would seem that the answer would depend on the degree of complexity that would have to be built into the parameter estimation program in order to obtain acceptable results. If it turns out that suboptimum methods of parameter estimation give results that are of practical utility, this will permit substantial savings in computation time.

REFERENCES

Adey, W. R., Kado, R. T., and Walter, D. O. (1967): Computer analysis of EEG data from Gemini flight GT-7. *Aerospace Medicine*, 38:345–359.

Bergland, G. D. (1969): A guided tour of the fast Fourier transform. *Institute of Electrical and Electronics Engineers Spectrum*, 6:41–52.

Bingham, C., Godfrey, M. D., and Tukey, J. W. (1967): Modern techniques of power spectrum estimation. *Institute of Electrical and Electronics Engineers Transactions on Audio Electroacoustics*, AU-15:56–66.

Blackman, R. B., and Tukey, J. W. (1958): *The Measurement of Power Spectra from the Point of View of Communication Engineering.* Dover Publishing Co., New York, 190 pp.

Cochran, W. T., Cooley, W. J., Favin, D. L., Helms, H. D., Kaenel, R. A., Lang, W. W., Maling, G. C., Nelson, D. E., Rader, C. M., and Welch, P. D. (1967): What is the fast Fourier transform? *Institute of Electrical and Electronics Engineers Transactions on Audio Electroacoustics*, AU-15:45–55.

Cooley, J. W., and Tukey, J. W. (1965): An algorithm for the machine calculation of complex Fourier series. *Mathematics of Computation*, 19:297–301.

Dumermuth, G. (1968): Variance spectra of electroencephalograms in twins. A contribution to the problem of quantification of EEG background activity in childhood. In: *Clinical*

Electroencephalography of Children, edited by P. Kellaway and I. Petersén. Almqvist & Wiksell, Stockholm, pp. 119–154.

Dumermuth, G. (1969): Die Anwendung von Varianzspectra für einen quantitativen Vergleich von EEG bei Zwillingen. *Helvetica Paediatrica Acta,* 24:45–54.

Dumermuth, G. (1970/71): Electronic data processing in pediatric EEG research. *Neuropädiatrie,* 2:349–374.

Dumermuth, G., and Flühler, H. (1967): Some modern aspects in numerical spectrum analysis of multichannel electroencephalographic data. *Medical and Biological Engineering,* 5:319–331.

Dumermuth, G., Huber, P. J., Kleiner, B., and Gasser, T. (1970): Numerical analysis of electroencephalographic data. *Institute of Electrical and Electronics Engineers Transactions on Audio Electroacoustics,* AU-18:404–411.

Dumermuth, G., Walz, W., Scollo-Lavizzari, G., and Kleiner, B. (1972): Spectral analysis of EEG activity in different sleep stages in normal adults. *European Neurology,* 7:265–296.

Gentleman, W. M., and Sande, G. (1966): Fast Fourier transforms—for fun and profit. *Proceedings of the Fall Joint Computer Conference,* pp. 563–578. *AFIPS Conf. Proc.,* Vol. 29. Washington, D.C. Spartan.

Kleiner, B., Flühler, H., Huber, P. J., and Dumermuth, G. (1970): Spectrum analysis of the electroencephalogram. *Computer Programs in Biomedicine,* 1:183–197.

Loomis, A. L., Harvey, E. N., and Hobart, G. A. (1937): Cerebral states during sleep as studied by human brain potentials. *Journal of Experimental Psychology,* 21:127–144.

Ormsby, J. F. A. Design of numerical filters with application of missile data processing. *Journal of the Association for Computer Machinery,* 8:440–446.

Rothman, J. E. (1968): The fast Fourier transform and its implementation. *Decuscope,* 7:3–10.

Schwartz, B. A. (1968): Afternoon sleep in certain hypersomnolent states: "intermediate sleep." *Electroencephalography and Clinical Neurophysiology,* 24:569–581.

Walter, D. O. (1963): Spectral analysis of electroencephalograms: Mathematical determination of neurophysiological relationships from records of limited duration. *Experimental Neurology,* 8:155–181.

Walter, D. O., and Adey, W. R. (1965): Analysis of brain-wave generators as multiple statistical time series. *Institute of Electrical and Electronics Engineers Transactions on Bio-Medical Engineering,* BME-12:8–13.

Walter, D. O., and Adey, W. R. (1966): Linear and non-linear mechanisms of brain-wave generation. *Annals of the New York Academy of Sciences,* 128:772–780.

Walter, D. O., Kado, R. T., Rhodes, J. M., and Adey, W. R. (1967): Electroencephalographic baselines in astronaut candidates estimated by computation and pattern recognition technique. *Aerospace Medicine,* 38:371–379.

Welch, P. D. (1967): The use of fast Fourier transform for the estimation of power spectra: A method based on time averaging over short, modified periodograms. *Institute of Electrical and Electronics Engineers Transactions on Audio Electroacoustics,* AU-15:70–73.

Automation of Clinical Electroencephalography.
Edited by P. Kellaway and I. Petersén.
Raven Press, New York © 1973.

Experience with Analysis and Simulation of EEG Signals with Parametric Description of Spectra

Lars H. Zetterberg

Royal Institute of Technology, Electrical Engineering Department, Telecommunication Theory, Stockholm 70, Sweden

I. INTRODUCTION

The conference in Houston on automation of clinical electroencephalography has given neurophysiologists and engineers an opportunity to discuss the objectives with automation, to report on the stage of development in methodology and to describe, by applications and examples, results achieved by the cooperation of these two groups. As one such example, I will describe some of the work that has been carried out in Stockholm by a group of doctors and engineers with members from the Department of Clinical Neurophysiology at the Karolinska Hospital and the Department of Telecommunication Theory at the Royal Institute of Technology (RIT). This work has been going on for several years and has been concerned with the development and clinical application of technical methods for analysis of EEG signals. The purpose is to extract information and to present it in a way that is convenient for neurophysiologists. The following two problems have guided the methodological work: spectral analysis of EEG signals with a computer and a parametric description of the spectral density, and detection of special wave forms such as spikes in an EEG signal.

The first issue has led to the development of computer programs for such an analysis, and this part of the work has been documented in several papers and reports, Zetterberg (1969a, b), Torstendahl (1969), and Andréasson

161

(1969). The clinical use of the method has begun, and a first report was given by Wennberg and Zetterberg (1971). In this report, some further results from two applications will be given: a study of a group of young healthy people (candidates to the school for Swedish Air Force pilots), and a study of a small group of patients with heart disease who have external pacemakers with a frequency that can be adjusted. In the present report, only partial results can be described; the complete reports will be given elsewhere.

The work on methodology and clinical applications has led to the development of some special equipment such as a correlator and a simulator of EEG signals (Zetterberg and Ahlin, *unpublished data*). Presently the group is engaged in making installation of equipment and computer programs at the Karolinska Hospital in order to facilitate the computer analysis of EEG in daily clinical work.

Work on the second issue has led to a computer program (Herolf, 1971) and also to the construction of equipment for carrying out the detection in analog form (see Zetterberg, *this volume*). The technique is being applied clinically, and work is going on to develop more general and effective computer methods.

In the present account, the application of the spectral analysis procedure on clinical cases has been emphasized, but it should be remembered that the situation is looked at from the point of view of an engineer. As background, the assumptions on which the analysis is based are stated. How the procedure is handled practically is described and illustrated. A way to describe an EEG spectrum by well-defined parameters is an essential result of our work. As a consequence, we have a method to simulate EEG signals which will be described. Experimentation with this equipment has given results that support the validity of our method of analysis.

II. METHODOLOGY

A. Parametric Description of the Spectral Density and the Autocorrelation Function

Correlation and spectral analysis of EEG signals constitute a well-established technique, and the theoretical basis for such an analysis is well known through works by Blackman and Tukey (1958), Blackman (1965), and Grenander and Rosenblatt (1956), among others. By taking the Fourier transform of the autocorrelation function (acf), or the autocorrelation coefficients (acc), the spectral density may be computed if certain precautionary measures are observed in order to secure reliable spectral estimates. The basic theory assumes stationariness of the observed process as a prerequisite to carrying out spectral analysis, but in a practical application it suffices if this is true during the observation time only. The question of stationariness for EEG signals is a debated topic in the literature. Some claim that it is stationary only during very short epochs of approximately 5 sec (Elul, 1968, 1969), whereas others regard approximately 20 sec as a reasonable length (Dumermuth, Huber, Kleiner and Gasser, 1971). We will come back to this question when discussing the results of our analysis of some clinical EEG registrations.

A characteristic of current methods for spectral analysis is that they require a fairly long registration time in order to get a good resolution in frequency and a good reliability in the spectral estimates, *i.e.,* a low statistical variability. This requirement will easily come into conflict with the assumption of stationariness for the EEG signals. In one way or another, one is forced to compromise, usually in terms of a moderate resolution in frequency and power density.

We have proposed a method for spectral analysis that may be interpreted as a further development of the correlation analysis. Instead of taking the Fourier transform of the observed correlation coefficients, they are used to estimate certain parameters in a function that is used as a model for the correlation function for a whole class of possible EEG signals. This function takes the form of a sum of exponentials and damped sinusoidals, as will be described. Instead of doing it directly, we prefer first to translate the model into the frequency domain and to state it in terms of spectral density.

It is assumed that the spectral density of an EEG signal, or rather a section of it, may be described by a rational function in the frequency variable f^2, *i.e.,* it is a function of the type

$$\frac{Q(f^2)}{P(f^2)} \tag{II-A-1}$$

where $P(x)$ and $Q(x)$ are polynomials in x with degrees p and q, respectively. In order to make the model attractive, it should be possible to keep p and q low, an assumption that experience confirms. In the majority of cases it is possible to take p and q less or equal to five. Typical values are $p = 3$, $q = 2$, and $p = 5$, $q = 4$.

A function of the form (II-A-1) allows resonances to appear in the spectral density, and it is possible to control both the resonance frequency, the bandwidth of a resonance peak and the power content related to a certain peak. In order to make these statements more precise, we perform a partial fraction expansion of (II-A-1), which allows the spectral density to be expressed as a sum of spectral components, each corresponding to one term in the fractional expansion. These terms appear to be of two types, depending upon where the poles or resonances are located. With type I, the poles are located on the negative imaginary axis in the s-plane ($s = \sigma + jf$), whereas for type II, the poles appear in conjugate pairs $\sigma \pm jf$ with $\sigma < 0$. Expressed in spectral density, the two functions are as follows:

$$\text{type I:} \quad R_{Ii}(f) = \frac{C}{f^2 + \sigma_i^2} \tag{II-A-2}$$

$$\text{type II:} \quad R_{IIi}(f) = \frac{Af^2 + B}{(f_i^2 + \sigma_i^2 - f^2)^2 + (2f\sigma_i)^2} \tag{II-A-3}$$

The first function has the resonance peak at $f = 0$, whereas the second has resonances close to $\pm f_i$ when σ_i is much less than f_i. The parameter σ_i measures the bandwidth of the resonance peak for type I and half the bandwidth for type II.

A weighted sum of terms of the stated types will give a function (II-A-1) where $q \leqslant p - 1$. If $q = p$, one more term is required which is a constant independent of frequency. We have called this a type 0 term (Wennberg and Zetterberg, 1971).

At this point it is convenient to translate the spectral functions back into the time domain by taking the Fourier transform. The result will be two types of correlation functions, called $r_I(\tau)$ and $r_{II}(\tau)$:

$$\text{type I:} \quad r_{Ii}(\tau) = G_i \exp\{-2\pi\sigma_i|\tau|\} \tag{II-A-4}$$

$$\text{type II:} \quad r_{IIi}(\tau) = (G_i \cos 2\pi f_i\tau - H_i \sin \pi 2 f_i|\tau|) \exp\{-2\pi\sigma_i|\tau|\} \tag{II-A-5}$$

The parameter G_i expresses the power contribution from each spectral component, whereas H_i gives a measure of the asymmetry for the spectral density relative to the resonance frequency f_i. The frequency parameters σ_i and f_i agree in the two sets of expressions, whereas the relations between G and H and the parameters A and B in the spectral density are somewhat involved (Zetterberg, 1969a, b).

In effect we have achieved a well-defined way to describe the spectral properties of an EEG registration by using certain frequency and power parameters. This way of presentation is illustrated in Figs. 1 and 2, which show how two typical EEG spectra may be built up from three spectral components. One of the components is of type I and two are of type II. The resonance frequencies for the latter are close to 10 and 20 Hz, and the peaks in the combined spectrum correspond to what is usually called α- and β-activity. The type I component has a bandwidth of 1–3 Hz, and it is conveniently identified with the δ-activity. For this reason it is appropriate to change the notation in order to facilitate the clinical use of our description system and analysis results (Wennberg and Zetterberg, 1971).

T5-OI / T6-O2

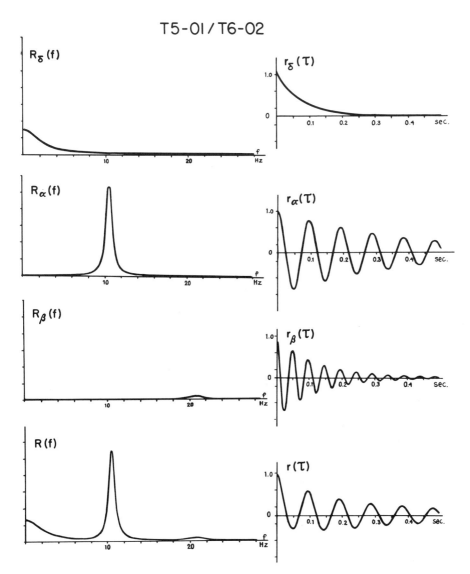

FIG. 1. Example of a composite EEG spectrum $R(f)$ built up as a sum of three components labeled $R_\delta(f)$, $R_\alpha(f)$ and $R_\beta(f)$. The corresponding autocorrelation functions are shown normalized.

F7-T3 / F8-T4

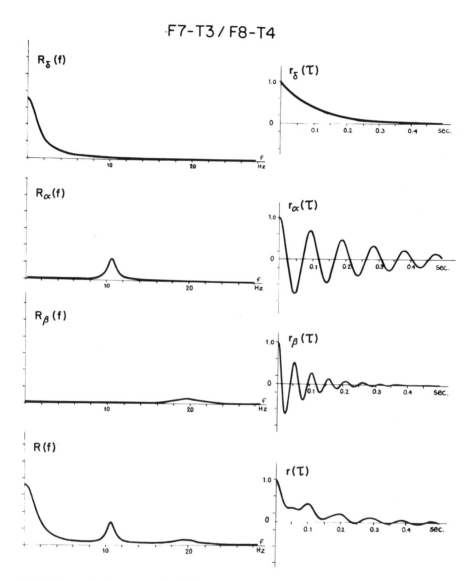

FIG. 2. Example of a composite EEG spectrum $R(f)$ built up as a sum of three components labeled $R_\delta(f)$, $R_\alpha(f)$ and $R_\beta(f)$. The corresponding autocorrelation functions are shown normalized.

δ-activity (type I):   frequency parameter σ_δ
                          power parameter G_δ

α-activity (type II):   frequency parameters σ_α, f_α
                          power parameters G_α, H_α

β-activity (type II):   frequency parameters σ_β, f_β
                          power parameters G_β, H_β

The total spectral density may be written

$$R(f) = R_\delta(f) + R_\alpha(f) + R_\beta(f) \qquad \text{II-A-6}$$

For this typical situation it suffices with 10 parameters to describe the EEG spectrum, which is indeed a very compact representation. In some cases we have found that the β-component is absent, and in some other cases it should be replaced by a ϑ-component with $0 < f_\vartheta < f_\alpha$. Examples of this situation are discussed below in the clinical cases. In a few exceptional cases it is necessary to add one more component, with a center frequency higher than f_β. This necessity has occurred when registrations are taken from patients for whom diazepam (Valium) has been prescribed. However, these results should be considered tentative.

In conclusion a model is set up for describing the spectral density and correlation function of an EEG signal. We believe that it may be used to define what should be meant by δ-, α-, β- and ϑ-activity by referring to the spectral components that have been introduced.

B. The Analysis Procedure

The model that was introduced to describe the spectral density and the acf is not convenient for setting up algorithms to carry out the computer analysis. Instead, another model is introduced that describes the sampled EEG signal $\{x_\nu\}$ in the form of a linear difference equation of order p:

$$x_\nu + a_1 x_{\nu-1} + \ldots + a_p x_{\nu-p} = e_\nu + b_1 e_{\nu-1} + \ldots + b_q e_{\nu-q} \qquad \text{(II-B-1)}$$

with $q \leq p$. The variables $\{e_\nu\}$ may be interpreted as an input sequence and the equation as a filter that transforms the input sequence into the output sequence $\{x_\nu\}$. In order to carry out the analysis it is convenient to make the assumption that the $\{e_\nu\}$ are uncorrelated and have a normal distribution with zero mean and variance γ^2. With this specification the process may be shown to be Gaussian and to have a rational spectral density of the form (II-A-1). To show this, the time-discrete representation must first be translated into a time continuous form and the parameter vectors $\bar{a} = (a_1, a_2, \ldots a_p)$ and $\bar{b} = (b_1, b_2, \ldots, b_q)$ must be expressed in terms of frequency and power parameters. This is described by Zetterberg (1969a, b), Torstendahl (1969) and Andréasson (1969), but it may also be established by a technique suggested by Gold and Rader (1969, ch. 3).

The assumption of normality has been introduced in order to derive an algorithm for estimating the parameter vectors $\bar{a}$ and $\bar{b}$ and to derive formulas for the statistical uncertainties in these estimates. It may seem to be a very specific assumption, since it is not true in general that an EEG signal has not even a first-order normal distribution (Saunders, 1963, 1967; Campbell, Brower, Dwyer and Lago, 1967; Elul, 1969). However, published results and our measurements show that the distribution is most often fairly close to a normal distribution when the observation time is approximately 20 sec. For longer times it is necessary to take into account time variations in the spectral power. Moreover, there are good reasons to believe that the assumption of normality is not critical for the estimation algorithm since it involves minimization of a function $Q(\bar{a}, \bar{b})$ that is quadratic in the observed variables $\{x_\nu\}$ with $\bar{a}$ and $\bar{b}$ as parameters. Such a function is reasonable also when the $\{x_\nu\}$ are not normally distributed. Finally, the validity of our model depends upon the results achieved and how meaningful they are. It must be emphasized that the mathematical model (II-B-1) is strictly a way of describing certain properties of an EEG signal, in particular its spectral density. It is not a model for the physiological generation of EEG signals.

The present procedure in analyzing EEG signals is first to select sections that are free from artifacts when judged visually. By artifacts we here mean pulses and disturbances such as spikes and muscular activity. Each section is divided further into segments of 10- or 20-sec length at the same time as sampling is carried out with a frequency of 200 Hz followed by A/D-conversion. One hundred acc are calculated for each segment. Estimation of the parameters is carried out in two steps. First the function $Q(\bar{a}, \bar{b})$ is minimized in the vector variables $\bar{a}$ and $\bar{b}$ taking into account certain restrictions to secure that Eq. (II-B-1) represents a stable filter. As a result, estimates $\bar{a}$ and $\bar{b}$ are achieved and also an estimate of γ^2. In the second step, these estimates are translated into estimates of the frequency and power parameters. At the same time the acc and the spectral density are calculated from these parameters and a comparison is made between estimated and measured autocorrelation coefficients. A detailed account of the estimation algorithm is contained in the report by Torstendahl (1969).

The estimation program is contained in a package that also includes a program for calculating the expected statistical uncertainties in the estimated parameters. Usually it is sufficient to write out the standard deviations for each parameter, but if desired, the complete covariance matrix may be displayed. The theoretical background is described by Zetterberg (1969a, b), and the complete program is described by Andréasson (1969).

Much more could be said about methodology and the measures that may be taken to improve performance. One essential parameter is the sampling rate, since it strongly affects the expected statistical uncertainties. We have found it convenient to use a mixed sampling scheme; that is, the mathematical model (II-B-1) is formulated for a sampling rate $f_m = f_s/s$, whereas the signal is sampled with the rate f_s. Usually f_s is taken to be 200 Hz and $s = (\text{step}) = 3$. Hence, only each third of the acc is actually being used for estimation purpose. Furthermore it is found convenient to premultiply the experimentally calculated acc with a function of the form $\exp\{-2\pi\mu|\tau|\}$ with $\mu = 0.5$ Hz. This measure improves the possibility to find the minimum of the function $Q(\bar{a}, \bar{b})$ in particular when α-activity is very stable in frequency or when there are tendencies of moderate nonstationarities in the recorded signal.

The analysis program is presently implemented on an IBM 360/75 and it takes typically 15 to 20 sec to carry out estimation and error analysis for each segment of EEG registration. Recently the estimation part of the program has been implemented on an IBM 1800 that is installed at the Karolinska Hospital (Stockholm), and equipped with a core memory of 32K. At the same time an installation is made at the department for Clinical Neurophysiology which includes a digital correlator specially designed for the purpose, a buffer memory, a computer interface, a punch unit with a paper tape punch and a paper tape reader. The correlator is connected with the computer through a local telephone cable, and it is now possible to calculate in real time the acc for a long registration and store it in the computer memory. The analysis must, however, be carried out off line. The paper tape unit allows each set of acc to be punched on paper tape and filed at the clinic. At a convenient time this set of acc may be read from the tape and transmitted to the computer. It may be remarked that preprocessing of the EEG which here results in a set of correlation coefficients simplifies the transmission and storage of EEG information.

C. Examples of EEG Analysis

In order to demonstrate the analysis procedure and the presentation of results, three examples of EEG analysis are displayed in Figs. 3–5. Each figure contains 10 sec of registration which equals half the registration being analyzed. The estimated parameters are displayed below each EEG signal, and they are grouped together in δ-, α- and β-components. The frequency parameters $\sigma_\delta, f_\alpha, \sigma_\alpha, f_\beta$ and σ_β are given in Hertz units, whereas the power parameters are in percent of the total power. The next line contains the calculated standard deviations of the estimated parameters with the same units being used. The interpretation is that these deviations will appear if a

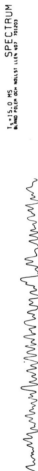

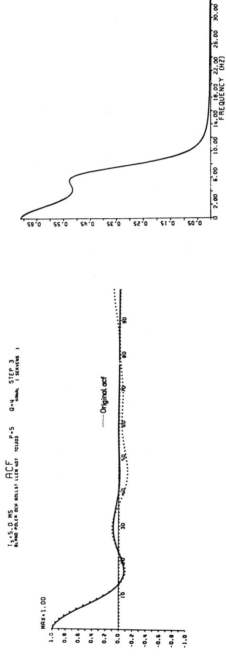

FIG. 3. Example of EEG signal analysis showing 10 sec of registration and estimated parameters with calculated standard deviations. One diagram shows autocorrelation coefficients determined from the recording and the autocorrelation function determined from estimated parameters. The other diagram shows estimated spectral density.

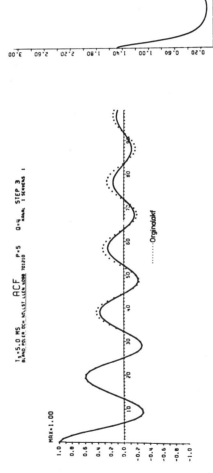

FIG. 4. Example of EEG signal analysis showing 10 sec of registration and estimated parameters with calculated standard deviations. One diagram shows autocorrelation coefficients determined from the recording and the autocorrelation function determined from estimated parameters. The other diagram shows estimated spectral density.

σ_δ	F$_\delta$%	f$_\alpha$	σ_α	G$_\alpha$%	H$_\alpha$%	f$_\beta$	σ_β	G$_\beta$%	H$_\beta$%
1.49	50	10.40	0.87	24	-1.5	19.78	0.77	27	0.8
± 0.08	7	0.05	0.05	4	1.5	0.04	0.04	4	0.8

1 S

T$_s$=5.0 MS ACF P=5 Q=4 STEP 3
BLAND POLER OCM NOLLST LLEN VISB 701210 NRWG. 1 SEKVENS 1

MAX=1.00

........Orginalacf

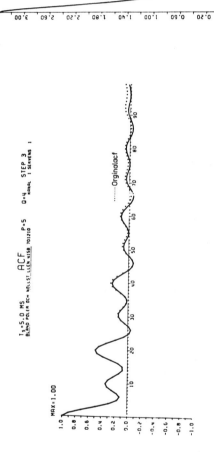

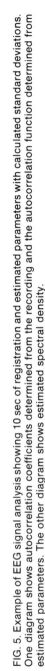

FIG. 5. Example of EEG signal analysis showing 10 sec of registration and estimated parameters with calculated standard deviations. One diagram shows autocorrelation coefficients determined from the recording and the autocorrelation function determined from estimated parameters. The other diagram shows estimated spectral density.

normal process is analyzed repeatedly for non-overlapping intervals, and this process has as parameters exactly those estimated out of the true EEG signal. It is likely that standard deviations for a true EEG signal will be larger than the computed ones. The figures also contain diagrams of the acc calculated from experimental data (dots) and of the acf (lines) calculated from estimated parameters. Finally, the calculated spectral density is displayed.

As can be seen, the EEG signals in the three examples are quite different. In Fig. 3, the low frequencies dominate; in Fig. 4, the α-activity is clearly visible, whereas Fig. 5 contains much high-frequency activity. These qualitative judgments can be made precise by looking at the estimated parameters. In Fig. 3 no statistically significant β-activity is found, whereas the δ- and α-activities have about 50% each. Notice that f_α is so low that the α-component could be called a ϑ-component. The statistical uncertainty is considerable for the power parameters $G_\delta (= F_\delta)$, G_α and H_α, whereas the estimated frequency parameters are much more precise, a conclusion that is valid in general. The analysis in Fig. 4 shows that the α-activity, i.e., the α-component, contains approximately 60% of the total power, whereas the δ-component has 30 to 35% and the β-component approximately 4%. The large amount of low-frequency activity may be surprising for those who are used to looking at EEG curves, but the conclusion is plausible regarding the difficulty one has in observing visually this type of activity in the signal. Moreover, similar results are evident from the Fourier analysis of EEG signals carried out by Dumermuth (1968). The α-activity is quite stable in frequency since $\sigma_\alpha = 0.58$ Hz implies that the 3-dB bandwidth is approximately 1.2 Hz. At the same time the statistical uncertainty in f_α and σ_α is low, and we conclude that a resolution of this kind would be impossible to achieve with conventional spectral analysis if only a registration length of 20 sec is being used.

The EEG signal in Fig. 5 contains much high-frequency activity, and the analysis shows that approximately 27% of the power belongs to the β-component. Despite this, about 50% of the power is located at low frequencies, the δ-component. Notice that f_β is very close to $2f_\alpha$, which may suggest a harmonic relation. This subject is discussed by Wennberg and Zetterberg (1971).

The agreement between experimentally calculated acc and the reconstructed acf is good in all three cases, which indicates that the program has succeeded in finding a true minimum of the function $Q(a, b)$. The situation is not so favorable in every case, and it may be necessary to rerun the program with another starting vector b or other order parameters p and q. We now use an F-test to decide which order should be preferred, as will be discussed in section IV-B under clinical applications.

III. SIMULATION OF EEG SIGNALS

Neurophysiologists may doubt the validity and utility of the parametric description of EEG spectra and the underlying mathematical model. We have emphasized, however, that this is strictly a means of describing certain properties of an EEG signal that is free from artifacts. In this section, certain results are reported which have been achieved in simulating EEG signals by making use of our mathematical model (II-B-1). Hopefully this discussion will provide evidence of the validity of our analysis procedure.

The most direct way to simulate an EEG signal is to implement eq. (II-B-1) on a computer and take as input $\{e_\nu\}$ a true or pseudo random sequence of normal variables, a technique that was used in Zetterberg (1969b). However, it is much more convenient to have a piece of equipment that allows generation of the signals in analog form and permits them to be recorded with a regular encephalograph.

There are at least two possibilities for constructing an analog EEG simulator. One is established by translating the time-discrete equation into continuous form which in turn may be interpreted as a transfer function between the white noise input $e(t)$ and the output $x(t)$. There are known methods to synthesize a network given the transfer function. This method is quite general but impractical for clinical use.

The other technique for analog generation is to start from the expansion of the spectral density in spectral components, expression (II-A-6). Each component may be realized by a separate network of first or second order, and the outputs are added to form the complete signal. It is then necessary to have separate white noise generators for each filter that are uncorrelated with each others.

This method has the advantage that it allows independent control of the frequency and power parameters for each component, but it has a limitation in that the method is not quite general with regard to the values of H that it is possible to realize with a second order network. In practice, it has not been found to be a serious limitation. The restrictions are that

$$G_i \geqslant O; \; \sigma_i G_i \pm f_i H_i \geqslant O \tag{III-1}$$

A block diagram of the last type of simulator is found in Fig. 6. It contains four separate noise generators, each one connected to a balanced modulator and followed by a filter of active RC-type. The noise generators are identical and make use of Zener diodes. In order to achieve white noise at low frequencies, which is essential for the application, the balanced modulators are inserted to translate a part of the spectrum with constant spectral density down to low frequencies. This will overcome a deficiency in the

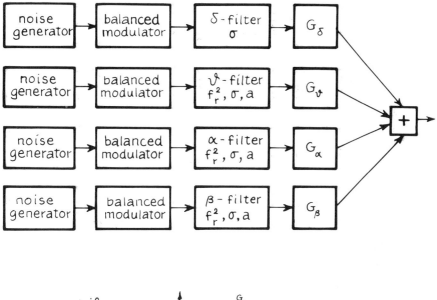

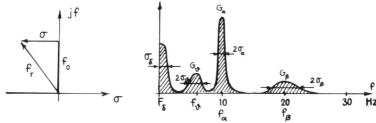

FIG. 6. Block diagram of EEG simulator realized with filters of active RC-type. Power parameters G are measured by connecting a power meter. Frequency parameters f_ϑ, f_α and f_β are labeled f_o and are controlled by f_r.

noise-producing properties of Zener diodes at these frequencies. The δ-filter is a first-order active RC-network, whereas the ϑ-, α- and β-filters are of second order. Potentiometers control independently the parameters f_r^2, σ and a where σ is the bandwidth parameter already introduced and f_r is related to the resonance frequency f_o as shown in the figure. The parameter a controls the zero of the transfer function, and thereby it is possible to set the power parameter H to a desired value within limits imposed by (III-1). The transfer function of the network may be written

$$H(s) = \frac{s + a}{(s + 2\pi\sigma)^2 + (2\pi f_o)^2} \qquad \text{(III-2)}$$

where σ and f_o are in Hertz units.

Figures 7 and 8 show two examples of true EEG signals and of the simulated versions where we have used the estimated parameters of the true EEG signal to set the parameters in the simulator. The registrations have been cut into convenient lengths of approximately 6 sec. In Fig. 7, there are six segments shown in the true EEG and four simulated ones, whereas Fig. 8 holds five of each. Can you classify them?

It has been found that the EEG simulator is most useful for testing the analysis program and the correlator that was mentioned in section II-B. The analysis program was discovered to be quite sensitive to quantization errors in the acc, i.e., to errors that are small but essentially independent from one coefficient to the next. Much greater precision is needed than the statistical errors may indicate since they appear as a result of a finite observation time. A quantization error not more than 0.5% is allowed when related to the largest value of $r(\tau)$, i.e., to $r(0)$.

We have also found it convenient to use the EEG simulator to create a catalog of typical EEG signals together with estimated parameters, acc and spectral density as shown in Fig. 3–5. We also think that an EEG simulator may be useful for educational purposes.

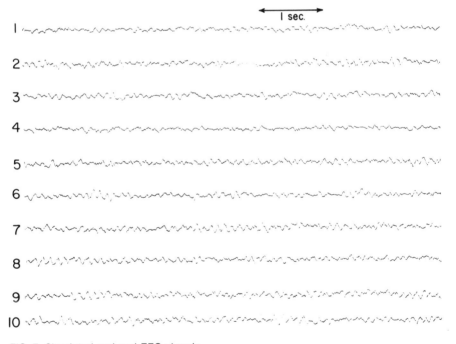

FIG. 7. Simulated and real EEG signals.

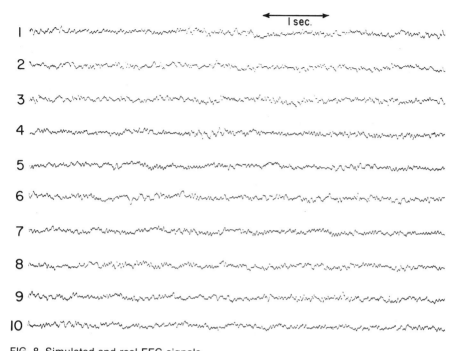

FIG. 8. Simulated and real EEG signals.

IV. EGG ANALYSIS APPLIED TO A GROUP OF
AIR FORCE CANDIDATES

A. Material and Analysis Procedure

The study concerned a group of candidates to the school of Swedish Air Force pilots, and the purpose was twofold. The first was to test our analysis procedure in a group of subjects in order to gain experience and to establish its performance characteristics. Essentially, Wennberg and Zetterberg (1971) achieved this purpose. That part of the study covered 25 of the candidates whose EEGs were all classified as normal on the routine visual examination. Certain statements could be made about typical parameter values and the variability within the group. Possible relations between parameters were investigated which led to interesting observations, e.g., about the relation between f_β and f_α. The second purpose of our study was to examine possible relations between the EEG parameters and the performance variables that are available. Or, stated in another way, are there any characteristics among the EEG parameters that relate to successful or unsuccessful behavior? For this purpose we selected 66 candidates who had finished school and passed examinations. Later, school grades and judgments were added to their files as well as the results of certain psychological tests and information about crashes and near-accidents together with a malfunction index. The later part of the study is presently being carried out by making a latent profile analysis on the EEG parameters.

Two series of registrations have been made. During the first one, the candidates were awake with closed eyes and they were sitting in a semi-reclining position. The same conditions applied during the second series, but stimulation with stroboscopic flicker was added. We call the two series "rest" and "stimulation," respectively. Flicker stimulation was carried out for a series of frequencies with nominal values 3, 10, 5 and 15 Hz, in that order. These measurements were made in succession with 20 sec for each frequency.

Electrode positions according to the 10–20 system were used, and the following channels were selected for computer analysis:

rest   F7–T3 and F8–T4
         T3–C3 and C4–T4
         T5–O1 and T6–O2

stimulation   C0–O1 and C0–O2

The recordings were written out on paper tape and scanned for artifacts. Sections free from artifacts were chosen with a length varying between 40 and 140 sec for the rest condition. The analysis was normally carried out with 20-sec segments; i.e., a succession of intervals were analyzed. In most cases, three to five segments were achieved in the rest condition; for certain individuals, there were six or seven segments, and for a few individuals only two segments could be used. For troublesome cases, analysis was carried out also with 10-sec segments.

An Elema-Schönander 16-channel electroencephalograph was used with a low-pass filter whose cut-off frequency was 30 Hz at 3 dB. Further details have been reported by Wennberg and Zetterberg (1971).

B. Survey of Analysis Results

A total of 1,699 segments have been analyzed by computer, of which the majority have a length of 20 sec. Most of the 10-sec intervals were used in connection with flicker stimulation. A preliminary study included repeated runs of analysis carried out on most intervals in order to find out which combination of parameters p and q gave the best agreement between experimental data and estimated parameters. First analysis was carried out with $p = 3$ and $q = 2$, but in most cases $p = 5$ and $q = 4$ were also used. The deviation between the experimentally determined acc and the reconstructed coefficients were examined and related to the statistical variability that the EEG acc are expected to show. This variability was calculated as a standard deviation for large arguments τ and for a process defined by the estimated parameters. If the deviation was found to be less than 1.5 times the calculated variability of the acc, the fit was judged to be good. If neither parameter combination gave such a fit, the analysis was continued with other parameter combinations, the selection of which was guided by plots of the autocorrelation coefficients.

With these results available from the computer analysis, an F-test was applied to select the best parameter combination (Scheffé, 1967; Kendall and Stuart, 1967; and Åström, 1967). In order to describe how this test is applied, it is convenient to introduce certain notations. Let $r = p + q + 1$, which is the number of parameters in our model that must be estimated. N denotes the number of samples that are taken, and γ^2 is the variance of the stochastic variables $\{e_\nu\}$ in Eq. (II-B-1). Let $\hat{\gamma}^2$ be the estimated value. A test is carried out between two models, denoted by index i and j with $r_i < r_j$, and the test variable is

$$\xi_{ij} = \frac{\hat{\gamma}_i^2 - \hat{\gamma}_j^2}{\hat{\gamma}_j^2} \cdot \frac{N - r_j}{r_j - r_i} \qquad \text{(IV-B-1)}$$

It is F-distributed with parameters $r_j - r_i$ and $N - r_j$. Since N is a large number — 4,000 for 20-sec registration — it is possible to use a table for $F(n_j - n_i, \infty)$. The following table is an extract for $r_j - r_i = 4$ that shows the relation between test variable and significance level. It applies when $p = 5$, $q = 4$ is being tested against $p = 3$, $q = 2$.

ξ	Significance level (%)
1.94	10
2.37	5
2.79	2.5
3.32	1
3.72	0.5
4.62	0.1

A study has been carried out to find if and how a certain value of the test variable relates to the agreement between experimental and reconstructed acc. In general it has been found that a large ξ is combined with a better approximation with model j than with model i, $j > i$, and the study has led us to accept 1% as the critical level; i.e., the chance is less than or equal to 1% that the model with index j will be preferred when the model with index i is really the true one.

Table 1 contains a survey of the results. It shows for different channels and for different values of p (and q) how many segments of analysis have been judged to give the best fit for that particular value. For each order p, column three labels the spectral components that the program gives as a result. For example, with $p = 3$, the result is one δ-component and either one α- or one β-component. Although there are three possibilities for $p = 4$ — namely, one α- and β-component or two δ-components and either one α- or one β-component — the computer program decides which combination gives the best fit.

TABLE 1. Survey of analysis results for Air Force candidates. Number of sequences for different orders. The total sum is 1699 sequences.

Order		Components	Rest			Stimulation
			T5–O1	F7–T3	T3–C3	C0–O1
p	q		T6–O2	F8–T4	T4–C4	C0–O2
1	0	δ	10	56	55	1
2	1	α or β	6	4	2	37
3	2	$\delta + \alpha$ or $\delta + \beta$	280	142	142	272
4	3	$\alpha + \beta$	3	0	0	15
4	3	$\delta + \delta + (\alpha \text{ or } \beta)$	6	6	2	4
5	4	$\delta + \alpha + \beta$	215	51	94	239
analysis unsuccessful			6	7	21	23
Sum			526	266	316	591

The third and fifth order systems obviously dominate Table 1, but a substantial number of segments for F7–T3, F8–T4 and T3–C3, T4–C4 lack any significant α- or β-component and therefore have only a δ-component, which is rather remarkable. The computer program has found a δ-component in almost all segments, and the exceptional cases occur mostly with flicker stimulation. A closer examination of these cases show that the α- or β-component has such a large bandwidth that its spectral density also covers low frequencies, and furthermore, that the center frequency is often so low that the α-component should rather be called a ϑ-component. We will see examples of this when flicker stimulation is discussed in more detail in the next section. Computer analysis has failed in approximately 3% of the cases, i.e., the algorithm has not found a minimum within the acceptable region of parameter values or the fit between original and reconstructed acc is not acceptable. These cases may indicate that the recordings have not been sufficiently stationary.

Typical estimated parameters are shown in Table 2 together with the calculated standard deviations. They represent mean values for 25 of the 66 candidates and are essentially an extract from Wennberg and Zetterberg (1971). The diagrams in Fig. 1 and 2 are based on these estimated parameters with H_α and H_β put equal to 0.

TABLE 2. Mean values of estimated parameters and calculated standard deviations for a normal group of young male adults

Parameter	T5–O1 T6–O2	F7–T3 F8–T4
Estimates		
σ_δ	2.2 Hz	1.5 Hz
G_δ	32%	67%
f_α	10.5 Hz	10.5 Hz
$2\sigma_\alpha$	0.85 Hz	1.25 Hz
G_α	58%	20%
f_β	20.7 Hz	19.4 Hz
$2\sigma_\beta$	2.6 Hz	4.0 Hz
G_β	4.5%	12.5%
S.D.		
f_α	0.1 Hz	0.36 Hz
f_β	0.36 Hz	0.52 Hz
$\sigma_\delta, \sigma_\alpha, \sigma_\beta$	25%	25%
G_δ	7% units	10% units
G_α	10% "	5% "
G_β	1% "	3% "

C. Influence of Stroboscopic Flicker on EEG Parameters

Figures 9–13 illustrate the information that the estimation program can produce, including plots of frequency and power parameters for five individuals for both left and right channels. The abscissa shows time scale in seconds, and as mentioned earlier, the nominal flicker frequencies have been 3, 10, 5, and 15 Hz, in that order. However, the actual frequencies have been slightly different, and it has been possible to determine these from the recordings, except for the individual F13:6 in Fig. 9. These frequencies are stated in the diagrams. For the diagrams that display frequency parameters, Figs. 9a–13a, the following variables are shown in Hz units: $\sigma_\delta, f_\alpha \pm \sigma_\alpha$ and

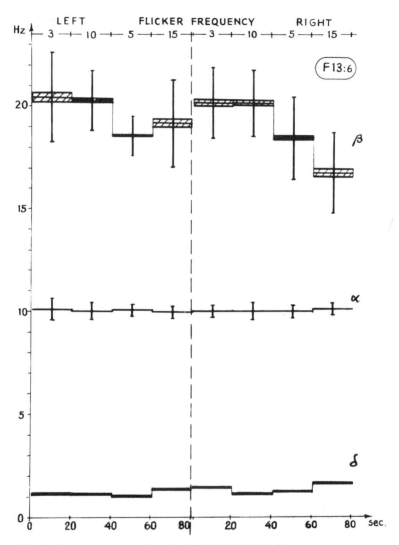

FIG. 9a. Frequency parameters during flicker stimulation.

$f_\beta \pm \sigma_\beta$ with $2\sigma_\alpha$ and $2\sigma_\beta$ marked by vertical strokes. The diagrams also indicate the statistical uncertainties for σ_δ, f_α and f_β by displaying two times the calculated standard deviations by the width of a shaded area or by the thickness of the horizontal line for that segment. The power parameters G_δ, G_α and G_β are shown in Figs. 9b–13b expressed in mW for a load of 1 ohm. Hence the estimated relative power parameters have been recalculated in absolute terms.

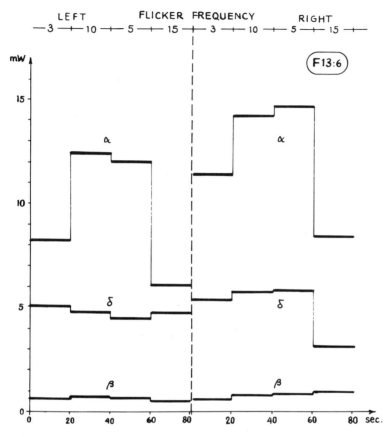

FIG. 9b. Power parameters during flicker stimulation.

From the diagrams we can see that people react in very different ways on flicker stimulation. Individual F13:6 is almost not affected at all in the frequency parameters and only moderately in the power parameters, whereas F30:6 and F19:4 (Figs. 12 and 13) show dramatic changes in their EEG parameters. In several instances there is a tendency for synchronism between flicker frequency and the resonance frequencies f_α and f_β; in particular, this is seen in Figs. 12 and 13, where f_α closely equals the flicker frequency for the second segment, but it is also seen in Fig. 10 (F23:2) where in the third segment f_α equals twice the flicker frequency. Furthermore, in Figs. 11 and 12, f_β equals the flicker frequency for the fourth segment, and it equals twice the frequency for the second segment in Fig. 11. Other tendencies to synchronism are also noticeable (for example, in Fig. 13), where for the third segment the α-activity is replaced by a broadbanded

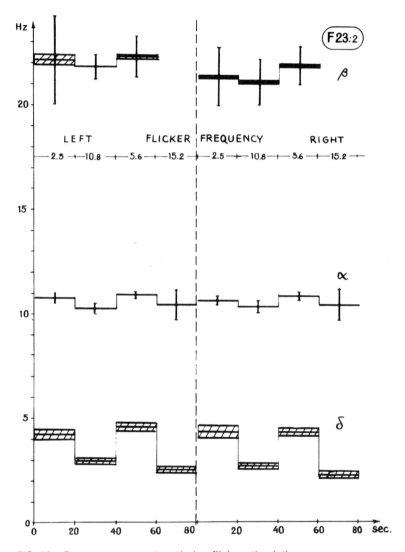

FIG. 10a. Frequency parameters during flicker stimulation.

ϑ-component with the center frequency equal to the flicker frequency. For the fourth segment in the same figure there is another example where a ϑ-component replaces the α-activity. For these two cases and one segment in Fig. 12, there is no δ-component but instead a broadbanded ϑ or β-component.

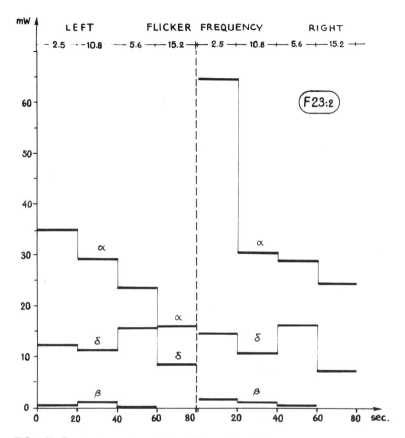

FIG. 10b. Power parameters during flicker stimulation.

If the diagrams for power parameters are scanned, considerable changes are observed from one segment to the next. However, we know from other measurements that large spontaneous changes often occur even in a rest situation. Furthermore, the statistical uncertainties are larger for the power parameters than for the frequencies. Hence, one should be cautious in looking for patterns in these diagrams. With these reservations let us point out that synchronization of f_α with the flicker frequency tends to decrease G_α (see Fig. 11, third segment; Figs. 12 and 13, second segment). It is gratifying to find that there is good agreement between estimated parameters for left and right channels for both frequency and power parameters, an indication that the analysis program gives meaningful results.

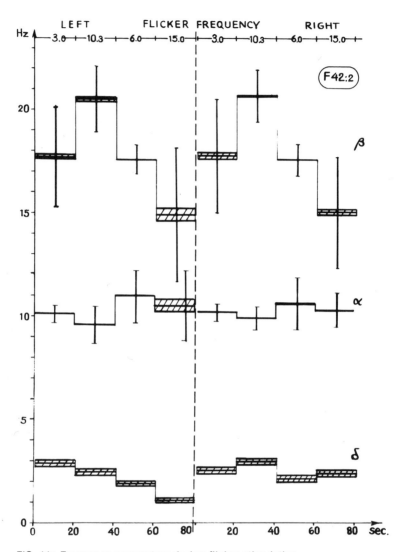

FIG. 11a Frequency parameters during flicker stimulation.

V. EEG ANALYSIS OF PATIENTS WITH EXTERNAL CARDIAC PACEMAKERS

It is reasonable to investigate if the EEG parameters may be used to detect physiological and psychological changes. The present study concerns a group of seriously ill cardiac patients who will eventually have pacemakers

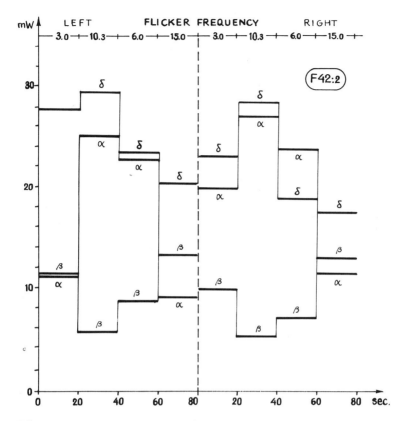

FIG. 11b. Power parameters during flicker stimulation.

implanted with fixed frequencies. During the investigation each patient had an external pacemaker with adjustable frequency. One purpose of the investigation was to find out which heart rate was best suited to each individual; this was determined by having the patient perform simple mental tasks with the pacemaker set to different heart rates. We then attempted to determine whether such changes would give rise to systematic changes in the EEG.

The patients sat with closed eyes, and periods of rest were alternated with test periods during which they performed simple arithmetic operations. The pacemaker was first set to a rate of 70 pulses/min, and the patient was at rest for 3 min, after which he performed a test lasting 40 to 80 sec, depending upon how quickly he carried out the arithmetic. The pacemaker was then adjusted to a new frequency, which took 1 to 2 min, and the patient was allowed 1 min of adaptation before the next rest and test sequence. During each such sequence, the EEG was recorded. The course of events

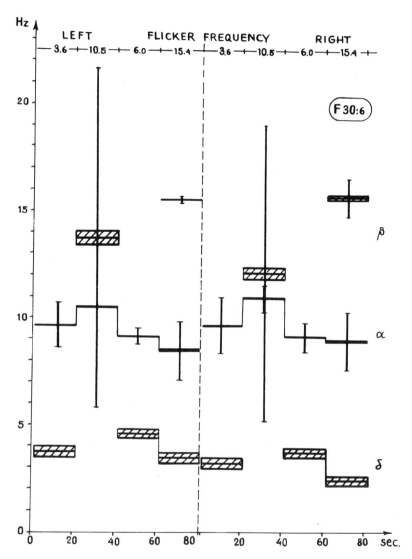

FIG. 12a. Frequency parameters during flicker stimulation.

was repeated for the following sequence of heart rates: 70, 55, 40, 70, 85, 100, and 70 pulses/min. For the last rate, no test was carried out. In all, the examination took approximately 45 min per patient.

Two series of experiments were performed on each patient. Before one series, the patient was given an experimental drug that is known from ani-

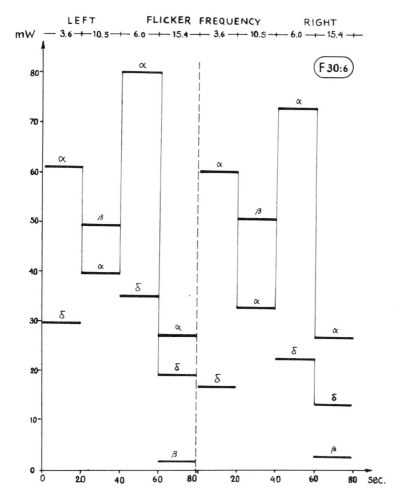

FIG. 12b. Power parameters during flicker stimulation.

mal experiments to protect the brain cells from a shortage of oxygen supply. It affects the DNA synthesis. Before the other experiment, only placebo was given. No member of the testing team knew when medicine or placebo was given. The medicine is new and not commercially available.

The account here has been somewhat sketchy but I hope it will suffice as a background for discussing the EEG analysis. Note that in these experiments there are several variables: the heart rate is changed, rest and test have been alternated and finally medicine and placebo are involved.

So far experiments have been carried out with 11 individuals, and re-

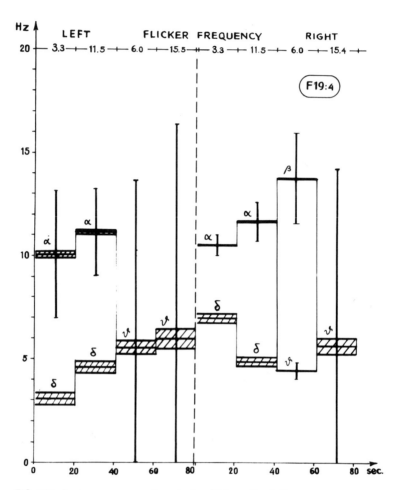

FIG. 13a. Frequency parameters during flicker stimulation.

sults from the EEG analysis are available for six persons. Two of these patients have been selected for the present study because the EEG computer analysis has given consistent and normal results. By this we mean that analysis has given the three components for δ, α and β with ordinary values of center frequency and bandwidth. In some cases no β-component has been found, but that, as we already know, is not an exceptional situation. Registrations from the two channels C3P3 and C4P4 have been analyzed with segments of 20 sec, which means that a consecutive sequence of nine segments is available in the rest condition and usually two or three segments during tests.

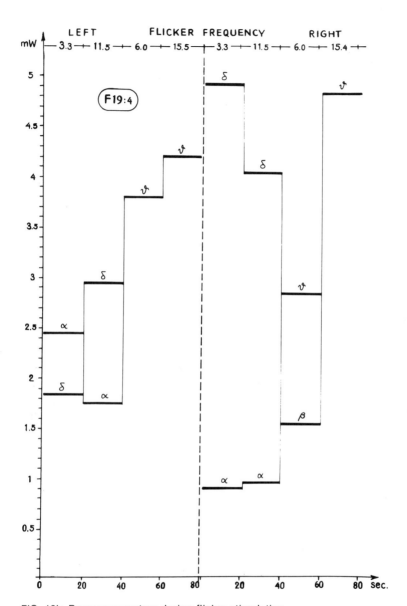

FIG. 13b. Power parameters during flicker stimulation.

First, diagrams were plotted that showed how frequency and power parameters changed from segment to segment, but these diagrams were difficult to survey. Next, average values were formed for each rest and test period. The results are shown in Figs. 14–17 and are organized as follows.

Patient	Experiment	σ_δ, f_α	G_δ, G_α	Treatment
		Diagram		
EG (male, age 67)	17:8	Fig. 14	Fig. 16a	medicine
	18:3	Fig. 14	Fig. 16b	plabo
PR (male, age 43)	23:3	Fig. 15	Fig. 17a	placebo
	24:3	Fig. 15	Fig. 17b	medicine

The power parameters G_δ and G_α have been handled in absolute power units and the diagrams separate results that refer to rest and test. They contain data both for left (C3P3) and right channels (C4P4). The sequence of heart rates has been stated already but they are only nominal values. Actual values differed somewhat from these and have been evaluated from the recordings. They are shown in each diagram. After the analysis had been carried out, information was given about which series was performed with the drug and which with placebo (see above).

Starting with the heart rate variable, results indicate that the frequency parameters σ_δ and f_α do not depend visibly on the heart rate within the range of variation. It is possible that the dynamics of the physiological reactions are so slow that definite changes did not have time to develop. The power parameters, in particular G_α, showed a large variation within each rest and test period, and therefore it is difficult to see any trends as a function of changes in heart rate. It is noticed that G_δ is in general more stable than G_α during a rest period.

When results are compared for rest and test periods, definite differences are observed. First, G_α decreased during test in all cases, which was an expected result, and at the same time G_δ increased, which is possibly a new result or at least less well known. The changes are considerable. The ratio of G_δ between test and rest are formed, and the same is done with G_α. We found that for G_δ, the ratio is approximately 2 and 2.3 for 17:8 and 18:3, whereas it is approximately 1.4 and 1.6 for 23:3 and 24:3. For G_α the ratio is 0.4 and 0.5 for 17:8 and 18:3 (*left*), whereas it is approximately 0.2 and 0.3 for 23:3 and 24:3 (*left*). Results indicate that it may be possible to use the ratio G_δ/G_α as an attention index. On the plots of parameters for each seg-

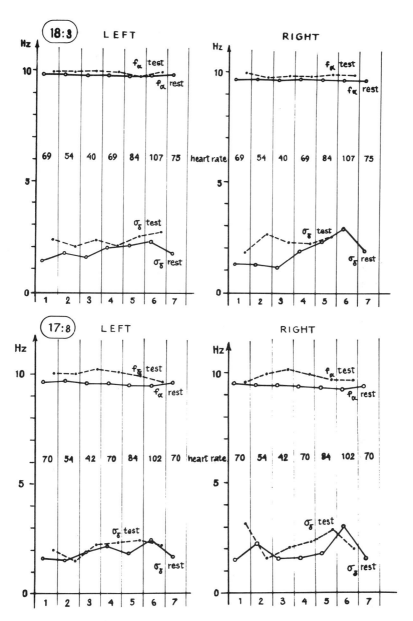

FIG. 14. Mean values of frequency parameters σ_δ and f_α during an experiment with a pacemaker patient in rest and test for different heart rates.

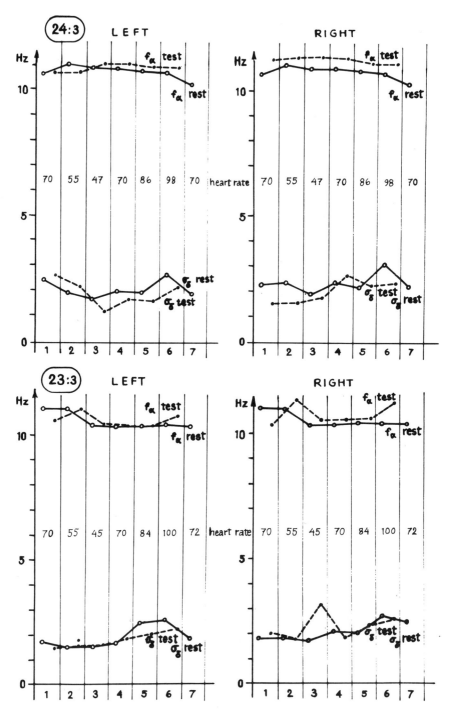

FIG. 15. Mean values of frequency parameters σ_δ and f_α during an experiment with a pacemaker patient in rest and test for different heart rates.

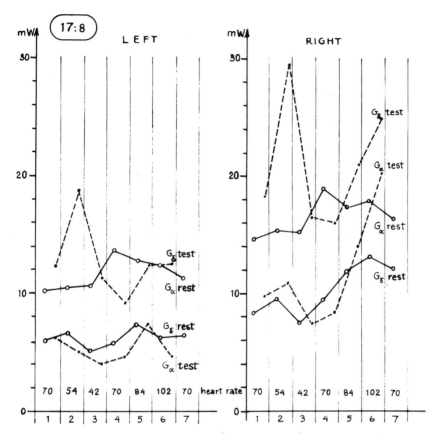

FIG. 16a. Mean values of power parameters G_δ and G_α during an experiment with a pacemaker patient in rest and test for different heart rates.

ment, it often occurred that G_α increased and G_δ decreased at the end of a test period, which may indicate a form of adaptation from test to rest.

When the diagrams of f_α are viewed, a difference is also here observed between rest and test situations. The frequency has a tendency to increase in the test situation and more so in those cases where the drug was given. The difference is then in most segments 0.5 Hz or more, which is highly significant. There are changes noticed with σ_δ, also, but the pattern is less clear.

VI. DISCUSSION AND COMMENTS

A model has been introduced for describing the spectral properties of an EEG signal with a set of frequency and power parameters. A method has been developed for estimating these from the recorded signal, and it has

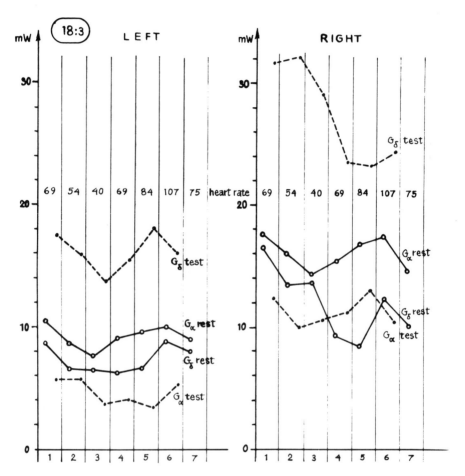

FIG. 16b. Mean values of power parameters G_δ and G_α during an experiment with a pacemaker patient in rest and test for different heart rates.

been tested on a large number of segments from EEG registrations. The results indicate that the method may be used to detect changes in the spectrum of an EEG signal as a result of stimulation by physiological and psychological means. These changes are given in quantitative form, and it also seems possible to detect small changes compared to what may otherwise be observed.

The model permits simulation of signals that closely resemble EEG signals, but there are of course characteristics of these that are not found in the simulated signals. That is the case with absence of symmetries in the amplitude distribution and the presence of special wave forms but also changes

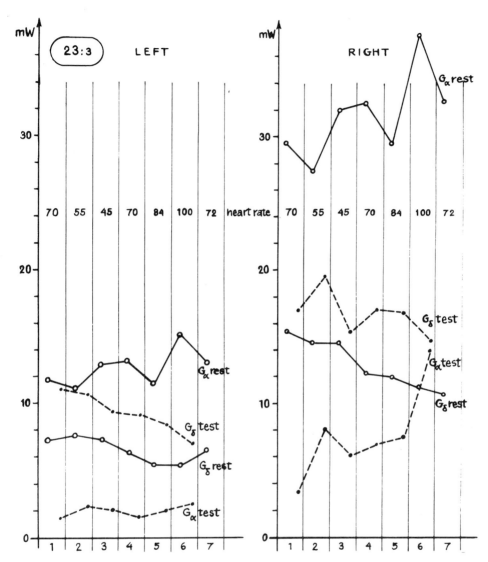

FIG. 17a. Mean values of power parameters G_δ and G_α during an experiment with a pacemaker patient in rest and test for different heart rates.

of the spectral properties with time. The last point is essential since it concerns in a fundamental way the assumption of stationariness that underlies the model. The parameters in our model are assumed to be fixed and independent of time during an observation interval of 10 or 20 sec, and this

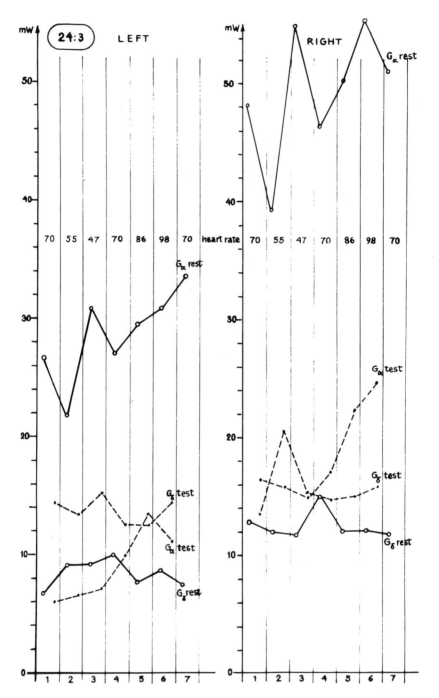

FIG. 17b. Mean values of power parameters G_δ and G_α during an experiment with a pace-maker patient in rest and test for different heart rates.

assumption implies that the observed process is stationary during that interval. Results show that it is a reasonable assumption for the frequency parameters, but it is less valid for the power parameters. We have observed in some cases such large changes in these parameters from one segment to the next that it is not reasonable to assume that they have been fixed during each segment. In particular this is true for the parameter G_α that measures that power in the α-component. It is lucky to observe that the analysis method gives meaningful results also in such a situation. By arguing heuristically it is seen that the estimation algorithm gives mean values of the power parameters during each segment, and with this interpretation results may still be used. However, as a consequence, the calculated statistical uncertainties in the parameters must be handled with caution, in particular for the power parameters.

Finally it may be mentioned that T. Bohlin (1971a, b) recently reported on a method for analyzing stochastic processes whose spectral properties change with time, slowly compared to the sampling frequency. He also uses a linear difference equation as a basic model but allows the coefficients in the left-hand side of (II-B-1) to change with time. At the same time he assumes a much larger order p than we do, and by this means it is possible to track changes in both frequency and power parameters. The analysis technique has been applied to a limited number of EEG signals, but very interesting results have been achieved in classifying EEG signals in the three categories "unchanging," "slow-changing" and "fast-changing."

ACKNOWLEDGMENT

Several people are involved in the work reported from the EEG group in Stockholm. On the clinical side, chiefly L. Widén and A. Wennberg have participated, whereas on the technical side, S. Torstendahl, I. Andréasson, K. Ahlin, A. Isaksson and the author have been involved with the spectral analysis issue. The group has been fortunate to cooperate with T. Bohlin, then at IBM Nordic Laboratory, Stockholm and now at RIT. He has extended the spectral analysis to cover also highly nonstationary situations (Bohlin 1971a, b). Spike detection has been worked on by M. Herolf and L.-Å. Dahlman on the technical side. The work presented in Section V was carried out in collaboration with Dr. K. Lagergren, Dept. of Psychiatry, Karolinska Hospital.

DISCUSSION

Discussion following Zetterberg's paper was concerned mainly with the significance and origin of relatively large amounts of energy in the delta range that have been evident in spectral profiles of the EEGs of normal human adults that have appeared in the literature. This type of spectral pattern is illustrated in Zetterberg's Fig. 4, where there is a substantial amount of activity seen below 2.0 Hz which is not clearly evident on visual examination of the relevant segment of EEG tracing.

Bickford reported (by letter) that the spectral analysis programs that he has been using on a PDP-12 computer in obtaining his compressed spectrograms do not show a large delta component (see Bickford, Fig. 2). He therefore questioned whether this delta activity is actually present in the EEG of most normal subjects or whether its appearance in some spectral analyses was an artifact of the computational techniques that had been used. Some of the discussants suggested that the absence of the delta components from Bickford's spectra might reflect particular features of Bickford's method of measurement and analysis. It was pointed out that Zetterberg had synthesized signals which had known spectral characteristics and which included a large "hump" in the delta range. A human electroencephalographer had not been able to detect that this was an artificial EEG signal and had not noted any visually detectable excess of delta components. Maulsby mentioned that he had used a Time-Data TD 100 for EEG spectral analysis and had found more delta activity than he would have expected from visual inspection of the relevant signals. He thought that this might have been due to DC offset at the time of starting the analysis equipment, since the delta "hump" was much higher when the analyses from short segments of EEG were averaged than when the analysis was performed on a relatively long section of EEG. Saltzberg suggested that folding of higher frequencies down into the delta range might account for the apparent large amount of delta activity, but he agreed with other discussants who considered that this was an unlikely explanation. Kellaway expressed the view that the delta activity was probably present in the normal EEG signal, but that it was not clearly evident because of superimposed rhythmic activity which was more obvious on visual inspection. In the very early days of life, the EEG has a large "baseline shifting," i.e., very low frequency oscillations of no fixed period. With increasing age we expect to see less baseline shifting and increasing superimposed theta, alpha, and beta frequencies. Electroencephalographers expect that there will be no baseline shifting in adults but in fact it is present. This baseline shifting is partly related to physiological state and is more marked when the eyes are closed than when they are open.

There was no generally acceptable explanation for this phenomenon, and Walter's comment that this was a problem "to let the specialists hassle about for a while" was the consensus of opinion considered on the matter.

REFERENCES

Andréasson, I. (1969): A computer program package for the analysis of a stationary process. *Technical Report No. 27, Telecommunication Theory.* Royal Institute of Technology, Stockholm.

Åström, K.-J. (1967): On the achievable accuracy in identification problems. *Proceedings of the IFAC Symposium in identification in automatic control systems, Prague paper 1.8.*

Blackman, R. B. (1965): *Linear Data-Smoothing and Prediction in Theory and Practice.* Addison-Wesley Publishing Co., Reading, Mass.

Blackman, R. B., and Tukey, J. W. (1958): *The Measurement of Power Spectra.* Dover Publications, New York.

Bohlin, T. (1971a): Analysis of stationary EEG-signals by the maximum likelihood and generalized least-squares methods. IBM Nordic Laboratory, *Technical Paper TP 18.200,* March 15.

Bohlin, T. (1971b): Analysis of EEG-signals with changing spectra. IBM Nordic Laboratory, *Technical Paper TP 18.212,* October 15.

Campbell, J., Brower, E., Dwyer, S. J., and Lago, G. V. (1967): On the sufficiency of autocorrelation functions as EEG descriptors. *Institute of Electrical and Electronics Engineers Transactions on Bio-Medical Engineering,* 14:49–52.

Dumermuth, G. (1968): Variance spectra of electroencephalograms in twins. In: *Clinical Electroencephalography of Children,* edited by P. Kellaway and I. Petersén. Almqvist & Wiksell, Stockholm, pp. 119–154.

Dumermuth, G., Huber, P. J., Kleiner, B., and Gasser, T. (1971): Analysis of the interrelations between frequency bands of the EEG by means of the bispectrum. A preliminary study. *Electroencephalography and Clinical Neurophysiology,* 31:137–147.

Elul, R. (1968): Brain waves: Intracellular recording and statistical analysis help clarify their physiological significance. In: *Data Acquisition in Biology and Medicine, Vol. 5,* edited by K. Enslein. Pergamon Press, Oxford, pp. 93–115.

Elul, R. (1969): Gaussian behaviour of the electroencephalogram: Changes during performance of mental task. *Science,* 164:328–331.

Gold, B., and Rader, C. M. (1969): *Digital Processing of Signals.* McGraw-Hill, New York.

Grenander, U., and Rosenblatt, M. (1956): *Statistical Analysis of Stationary Time Series.* Almqvist & Wiksell, Stockholm.

Herolf, M. (1971): Detection of pulse-shaped signals in EEG. *Technical Report No. 41, Telecommunication Theory.* Royal Institute of Technology, Stockholm.

Kendall, M. G., and Stuart, A. (1967): *The Advanced Theory of Statistics, Vol. 2.* Charles Griffin & Co. Ltd., London.

Saunders, M. G. (1963): Amplitude probability density studies on alpha and alpha-like patterns. *Electroencephalography and Clinical Neurophysiology,* 15:761–767.

Saunders, M. G. (1965): Amplitude probability density studies of alpha activity in the electroencephalogram. In: *Mathematics and Computer Science in Biology and Medicine,* Medical Research Council. Her Majesty's Stationary Office, London.

Scheffé, H. (1967): *The Analysis of Variance.* John Wiley & Sons, New York.

Torstendahl, S. (1969): A computer program for EEG analysis. *Technical Report No. 28, Telecommunication Theory.* Royal Institute of Technology, Stockholm.

Wennberg, A., and Zetterberg, L. H. (1971): Applications of a computer-based model for EEG analysis. *Electroencephalography and Clinical Neurophysiology,* 31:457–468.

Zetterberg, L. H. (1969a): Estimation of parameters for a linear difference equation with application to EEG analysis. *Mathematical Biosciences,* 5:227–275.

Zetterberg, L. H. (1969b): Analysis of a large-sample-procedure for estimating parameters in a linear difference equation. *Technical Report No. 26, Telecommunication Theory.* Royal Institute of Technology, Stockholm.

Automation of Clinical Electroencephalography.
Edited by P. Kellaway and I. Petersén.
Raven Press, New York © 1973.

Reverse Correlation Analysis of Slow Posterior EEG Rhythms in Adults

E. Kaiser, I. Petersén and R. Sörbye

Kaiser Laboratory, Copenhagen, Denmark, and Department of Clinical Neurophysiology, Sahlgren Hospital, Göteborg, Sweden

Rhythmical slow activity in posterior EEG leads has gained increasing attention during the last decade. A survey of such rhythms was presented by Aird and Gastaut (1959). Among the posterior rhythms, one was originally presented by Pitot and Gastaut (1956), and was also mentioned by Nayrac and Beaussart (1956) and by Vallat and Lepetit (1957). The rhythmic activity, the frequency of which is approximately 2.5–4.5 Hz and the voltage most often 40–50 μV, is usually bilaterally symmetrical; sometimes, however, it demonstrates a left-sided or, more often, a right-sided preponderance. Vogel and Götze (1959) noted that this activity was inhibited by arousal stimuli. Petersén and Sörbye (1962) observed that it disappeared in sleep. The slow rhythmic activity appears in less than 0.5% of normal adults (Selldén, 1964; Eeg-Olofsson, 1970). Kuhlo, Heintel and Vogel (1969) assumed a frequency between 0.025 and 0.075%.

In order to investigate the periodicity and the temporal pattern of such rhythms, a special method was introduced by Kaiser and Petersén (1965, 1966). This method, reverse correlation, was based on a convolution technique, similar to the standard autocorrelation (see Kaiser, Magnusson and Petersén, 1967). Equation (1) shows the reverse correlation and, for the sake of comparison, the autocorrelation (2).

203

$$g_{(1)} = \frac{1}{T} \int_{-\frac{T}{2}}^{+\frac{T}{2}} f_{(t+\frac{\tau}{2})} \cdot f_{(1-\frac{\tau}{2})} d\tau \qquad (1)$$

$$h_{(\tau)} = \frac{1}{T} \int_{-\frac{T}{2}}^{+\frac{T}{2}} f_{(t+\frac{\tau}{2})} \cdot f_{(1-\frac{\tau}{2})} dt \qquad (2)$$

The difference between the two operations appears in the way the convolution products are summed with respect to τ and t. The reverse correlation is a continuous function in time, whereas the autocorrelation can be regarded as the "summary" of periodic activities in the time interval T. All phase interrelations in the reverse correlation method are preserved, and changes in the temporal pattern (non-stationariness) are reflected in the output.

An extension in the convolution technique has been developed (Kaiser and Petersén, 1966) which implies simultaneous representation of the input data in two different time scales in the data window. By means of adjusting the ratio in the time scales, it is possible to penetrate the intercorrelations between two or more frequency components in the rhythmic activity.

The reverse correlation technique was used earlier in a restricted number of clinical materials only: by Kaiser and Petersén (1968) in a study of 14 and 6 Hz positive spikes in normal children, by Petersén, Hambert, Kaiser, Magnusson and Sörbye (1969) and by Hambert and Petersén (1970) in analyses of slow posterior rhythms in patients suffering from myoclonus epilepsy.

MATERIAL AND METHODS

EEGs were recorded from 40 patients showing slow posterior rhythmic activity in the frequency range 2.5–4.5 Hz (Fig. 1). A sampling period of 1 min was started at the onset of the first run of slow activity and consisted of at least six distinct slow waves in a series. The samples then were subjected to repeated reverse correlation analyses in the time scale ratios 1:1, 1:2, 1:3 and 1:2.5 (a1, b1, c1, and d1, respectively, in Fig. 2). In order to facilitate evaluation of the reverse correlation data, a subsequent reverse correlation analysis of the primary analysis data was performed in the analysis ratio 1:1 (a2, b2, c2, and d2, respectively, in Fig. 2). At the top of Fig. 2, the original EEG signal can be seen, including a 3.5 Hz rhythmic activity.

Further evaluation of the ink-recorded secondary analysis was based on visual determination of the appearance and the disappearance of each rhythmic sequence in the different ratios.

As described earlier by Kaiser and Petersén (1966), the analysis output

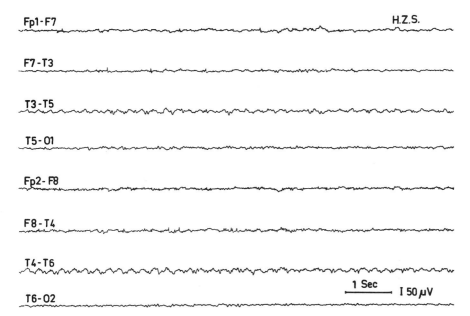

FIG. 1. Rhythmic 3.5 Hz activity in parieto-temporal leads, bilaterally synchronous and symmetrical, occurring in long series.

in the ratio 1:1 appears with frequencies two times the parent frequencies. In analysis ratios outside the range 1:1, the analysis output appears at frequencies equal to the sum of the parent frequencies. Consequently a second analysis in the ratio 1:1 will demonstrate an output frequency, which in the former case is four times the parent frequencies. In Fig. 2, a2, the parent frequency thus is one-quarter of the obtained a2 analysis output frequency. The parent frequencies f_x and f_y are obtained via the following equations:

$$f_x = f_2 \cdot \frac{0.5r}{1+r} \tag{3}$$

$$f_y = f_2 \cdot \frac{0.5}{1+r}, \tag{4}$$

where f_2 is the frequency of the secondary analysis output signal and r the chosen time-scale ratio.

For each patient, the epochs of rhythmic activity in a2–d2 were indicated by solid and broken lines, as in Fig. 3. In 1:1 the slow rhythmic activity epochs are symbolized by solid horizontal lines, which indicate the "on" time of the slow rhythmic frequency in the EEG, and the broken lines, which represent the fast rhythmic activity within the alpha range. In the ratio 1:2

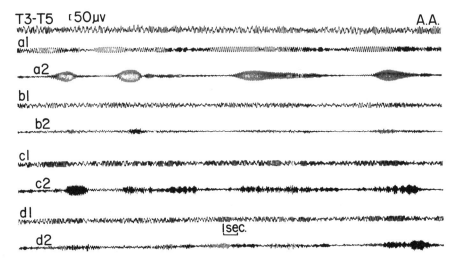

FIG. 2. Above the original EEG signals (T3–T5). Analysis on the ratio 1:1, 1:2, 1:3, and 1:2.5 (a1, b1, c1, d1) and subsequent re-analyses in ratio 1:1 (a2, b2, c2, d2) during a part of the analysis minute in one patient. The analysis output expresses at any time the instantaneous mean activity being derived in the data window; consequently, a noticeable delay is produced. In the present case, the window width is 2.5 sec, and the output-delay amounts to 1.25 sec, equal to half the window-width (curves a1–d1; see Kaiser and Petersén, 1966). In the case of a secondary analysis (a2–d2), the total delay is increased to 2.5 sec with respect to the primary signal.

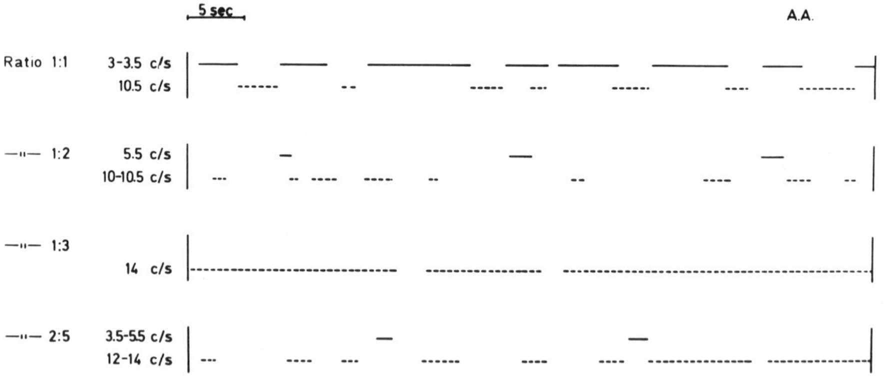

FIG. 3. Occurrence of various rhythmic activities in the different reverse analysis ratios during the total analysis minute in the same patient as that in Fig. 2.

the broken lines represent the fast rhythmic activity within the expected frequency range of an interference between the slow original rhythm and the doubled frequency of this, the solid lines indicating different subharmonics. Principally the same is to be said about the ratios 1:3 and 1:2.5 (in the present case no slow activity dominance is found in the 1:3 analysis ratio).

The data were expressed as the percentage time any rhythmic activity occurs as dominating activity or as activity possibly dominated by the fundamental activity. Fig. 4 shows an example of this treatment.

A further study of the temporal occurrence of the different rhythmic activities and their combination was established on the basis of punched cards carrying the individual data and a computer treatment of the total material. The rhythmic activities are numbered 1–8, numbers 1, 3, 5 and 7 indicating the slow rhythmic activity in ratio 1:1, 1:2, 1:3 and 1:2.5, respectively, and numbers 2, 4, 6, 8 indicating in the same way the fast rhythmic activities.

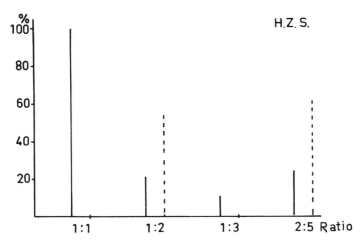

FIG. 4. Percentage of occurrence of different rhythmic frequencies during the analysis minute in the same patient as in Fig. 1.

RESULTS

Table 1, column 2, shows, in percentages, the occurrence of the 1 + 13 most frequently appearing combinations of activities (where the first combination indicates no activity). The composition of these combinations are seen in column 1. In 14.3% of the total time, no established rhythmic activity is found. Considering the occurrence of each rhythmic activity in the different combinations, the total appearance of every single type of rhythm is shown in the remaining columns in Table 1.

TABLE 1. Temporal activity distribution in B material
(selected for most frequent activity combinations)

Activity combinations	Time (%)	Occurrence of single activities (%)								
		0	1	2	3	4	5	6	7	8
–	14.33	14.33								
1	8.50		8.50							
1 + 5	3.50		3.50				3.50			
1 + 6	3.33		3.33					3.33		
2	3.33			3.33						
1 + 6 + 8	3.17		3.17					3.17		3.17
1 + 3 + 5 + 7	3.17		3.17		3.17		3.17		3.17	
1 + 3 + 7	2.83		2.83		2.83				2.83	
1 + 7	2.83		2.83						2.83	
2 + 6 + 8	2.67			2.67				2.67		2.67
1 + 4 + 8	2.67		2.67			2.67				2.67
7	2.50								2.50	
1 + 4 + 6 + 8	2.33		2.33			2.33		2.33		2.33
1 + 4 + 5	2.33		2.33			2.33	2.33			
Total %	57.49	14.33	34.66	6.00	6.00	7.33	9.00	11.50	11.33	10.84

When periods of no rhythmic activity were disregarded, the greatest probability (8.5%) for the single occurrence of low-frequency rhythm occurred in the analysis ratio 1:1. A number of temporal combinations of rhythms being all of nearly the same probability, 3.5–2.5%, are further shown in the table. In six combinations, the specifications express simultaneous occurrence of low-frequency rhythmic activity in the ratio 1:1 and 1:3. Single occurrence in the ratio 1:1 of high-frequency activity (alpha) was found in 3.3% of the recording time. Other combinations are more complicated.

Thus we find low-frequency rhythmic activity in the ratio 1:1 with simultaneous relatively high-frequency dominance in ratios 1:3 and 1:2.5. Low-frequency dominance in the ratio 1:1 is seen simultaneously with low-frequency dominance in the ratios 1:2, 1:3, and 1:2.5, sometimes the ratios 1:1 and 1:2.5 or the ratio 1:2.5 only. Further we see low-frequency dominance in the ratio 1:1 combined with high-frequency dominance in the other ratios.

Table 2 gives as a percentage the temporal occurrence of the different rhythmic activities numbers 1–8. A gives the percentage of distribution of these activities in the total material. B indicates the percentage of distribution of the same activities in the material explained in Table 1 (containing the 13 most common combinations of activities when zero-activity is omitted). C gives the percentage of distribution in the remainder of the total material when B is subtracted from A.

TABLE 2. Temporal activity distribution in A, B and C materials

Activity material	Occurrence of single activities (%)							
	1	2	3	4	5	6	7	8
A (total	62.52	16.39	18.64	21.48	16.65	29.50	23.78	23.55
B	34.66	6.00	6.00	7.33	9.00	11.50	11.33	10.83
C (A–B)	27.80	10.39	12.64	14.15	7.65	18.00	12.45	13.72

Table 2 shows that low-frequency activity in the analysis ratio 1:1 (activity 1) is the most common in the total material and in the selected material as well. High-frequency activity (activity 6) in the analysis ratio 1:3 appears at a time percentage next to activity 1. The other activities appear in percentage orders of only slight differences. The most marked difference between the B and C materials is seen in the activities 2, 3 and 4. Compared to the low-frequency activity in the ratio 1:1, only 17% is in the B material but nearly twice that amount in the C material. The same percentage interrelation appears when low-frequency activity and high-frequency activity in the ratio 1:2 are compared.

The interrelation in pairs of the rhythmic activities was investigated in the total material and in the selected parts of it as well. Two examples are shown in Fig. 5. Figure 5a shows the interrelation between the activities 5 and 6 (dominance of low and high frequency, respectively, in the ratio 1:3) in those 28 patients presenting these activities. The abscissa indicates the activity number 5 in percentage of the analysis minute. The ordinate indicates the activity number 6 in the same way. Analogously, Fig. 5b shows the interrelation between the rhythmic activities number 6 and 8 (high-frequency dominance in the ratios 1:3 and 1:2.5, respectively). In Fig. 5a, as well as 5b, the orthogonally determined regression line is drawn. In Fig. 5a, a regression coefficient of -1.22 and a correlation coefficient of 0.59 are found, which, with $N = 28$, gives a correlation on the 0.999 probability level. The negative interrelation between activities 5 and 6 indicates simply an expected complementarity regarding the dominance of high and low frequency activities in the 1:3 ratio. In Fig. 5b we find a regression coefficient of 0.65 and a correlation coefficient of 0.66 with $N = 34$, indicating correlation on

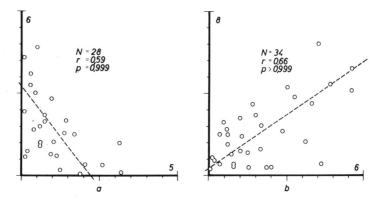

FIG. 5. Two examples showing the possible interrelation between the activity 5 and 6(a) and 6 and 8(b). In (a), a negative interrelation appears, whereas the interrelation in (b) is positive.

the same level. This correlation expresses a proportionality between high-frequency components in the ratio 1:3 and 1:2.5.

The regression lines as well as the correlation coefficients and the correlation probabilities, including the significance of these, have been estimated with regard to the possibilities of combination between rhythmic activities in pairs. One set of calculations has been carried out concerning the total material (Table 2, A), another set regarding the selected material of the 13 most commonly appearing combinations of activities (Table 2, B), and lastly one set concerning the remaining material (Table 2, C). Considering the distortion of the material coming out when any of the coordinates equals zero, the calculations of the regression and correlation coefficients have been carried out after excluding pairs of coordinates containing a zero value.

On the basis of the numbers of coordinate pairs in every calculation or correlation, the level of significance has been determined. Only values of correlation with significance at least of 90% have been included. Table 3 shows the regression coefficients with significant correlation regarding the total material. Every field has room for three numbers, of which the upper one shows the regression coefficient of the A material, the next number regarding the B material and the last one the C material. The values in parentheses indicate correlation probability between 90 and 95%; the others indicate a correlation probability of 95% or higher. The table shows, as expected, generally negative correlations between high and low frequency activity at the same analysis ratios, and positive correlations between low-frequency components and different analysis ratios.

TABLE 3. Significant interrelations (regression-coefficients) among activities 1–8

	H2	L3	H4	L5	H6	L7	H8
						4/1	4/1
L1	−0.72	(+0.41)	−	+0.41	−	(+0.53)	−
	−0.32	+0.82	(+0.23)	+0.59	−	+0.68	−
	−	+0.68	−	−	+0.73	+0.57	−
	LH	LL	LH	LL	LH	LL	LH
						4/1	4/1
H2		−	−	(−0.82)	−	−	+0.70
		−	−	−	+1.51	−	+1.29
		−	−	−0.78	−	−	+0.40
		HL	HH	HL	HH	HL	HH
						4/5	4/5
L3			(−0.92)	−	−	+1.29	−
			−	+0.65	(−0.28)	+1.09	−
			−	(−0.23)	+1.19	−	(+0.30)
			LH	LL	LH	LL	LH
						4/5	4/5
H4				−	−	−	−
				−	−	−	+2.16
				−	−	−	−
				HL	HH	HL	HH
						4/33	4/33
L5					−1.22	−	(−0.91)
					−0.59	(+1.72)	−
					−	−	−
					LH	LL	LH
						4/33	4/33
H6						−	+0.65
						(−4.03)	+0.92
						+0.61	−
						HL	HH
							4/4
L7							−0.94
							(−0.86)
							−
							LH

It is difficult to see a general pattern in the interrelation between high-frequency components in the different analysis ratios.

Table 4 shows that the A material includes 12 values indicating a correlation probability of 90% or more, seven of these with a level of 95% or more, four with a level of 99% or more, and three indicating a level of 99.9%. In the B material there are 16 values of correlation probability on the 90% level or more, of which 11 are at least on the 95% level, seven on the 99%

and three on the 99.9% level of probability. In the C material, nine values of correlation probability are on the 90% level or better, seven on the 95% level or better, four on at least a 99% level and one on the 99.9% level.

TABLE 4. Number of significant correlations on the 90, 95, 99 and 99.9% levels and their relation to expected number of correlations in random data (in parentheses)

Material	Level			
	90%	95%	99%	99.9%
A	12 (4.3)	7 (5.0)	4 (14.3)	3 (107.0)
B	16 (5.7)	11 (7.9)	7 (25.0)	3 (107.0)
C	9 (3.2)	7 (5.0)	4 (14.3)	1 (36.0)

Assuming the coordinate pairs of the 28 combinations occur at random, one would expect an average of 2.8 values regarding correlation probability of 90% or more, 1.4 values at the 95% level and 0.28 and 0.028 values at the 99 and 99.9% levels, respectively. In the A material, 12 correlations have been found at the 90% level. Compared to the expected value of 2.8 in random data, the actual number (12) is 4.3 times higher. Such ratios at the different probability levels in the three materials are given in Table 4 within parentheses adjacent to the number of significant correlation. From the table it is clear that the selected B material shows considerably higher correlation than the total material and, as one may expect, that there is a considerably lower correlation in the C material.

On the basis of the 1 + 13 most common combinations of rhythmic activities, we have investigated which sequential patterns appear most frequently. Choosing sequences of three, we found 19 characteristic different sequences which, in the total material of 2000 combinations, each recurred six to nine times. The most frequently recurring single rhythmic activity in these sequences was, as could be expected, low-frequency activity in the ratio 1:1. This activity was found in 14 of the 19 sequence patterns. The five remaining sequences were dominated by a high-frequency rhythmic activity in the ratio 1:1. The changes between activity combinations during the sequences were on an average two per sequence and were grouped as regards number of changes in the following way: no changes in the ratio 1:1, some changes in the ratio 1:2, greater changes in the ratio 1:2.5, and the greatest changes in the ratio 1:3.

DISCUSSION

The small representation of the activities 2, 3 and 4 in the B material compared to the representation of these activities in the C material expresses that the high-frequency activity in the ratio 1:1 in the B material has a rather low representation. The same is true in the B material concerning the analysis ratio 1:2. This finding may indicate that small alpha wave amplitudes, possibly combined with low second subharmonic activity, may give rise to recurrent appearance of the activity patterns characterizing the B material. Initially we assumed that the appearing harmonic interrelations in the ratios 1:2 and 1:3 indicated the low-frequency components in the posterior slow waves as subharmonics to the alpha waves; hence it was surprising to notice that interrelated rhythms appeared more frequently in the ratio 1:2.5 (activity 7 and 8) than in the ratios 1:2 and 1:3 (activities 3-4 and 5-6, respectively). The established interrelations therefore cannot be explained as *simple* subharmonics to the alpha waves. This obviously is in accordance with the observation in one patient by Kuhlo (1967), who found an alpha frequency of 8-9 Hz 18 days after an accident and 10-11 Hz a year later, the 4-5 Hz rhythm remaining unchanged.

We will mention two possible explanations of our findings.

(1) *The low-frequency rhythmic activity is driven by alpha waves or is driving the alpha waves in a harmonic pattern.* The interaction between neuronal generators of different frequencies is assumed on the basis of nonlinear interneuronal transmission. The tidal possibility for interaction in a rhythmic pattern is considered to be confined to moments of certain fixed-phase interrelations. In rhythms having a frequency interrelation in the ratio 1:2, identical phase interrelation occurs one time per period, viewed from the low-frequency generator, and one time per two periods, viewed from the higher frequency generator. In the frequency ratio 1:2.5, the same phase interrelation occurs one time in two slow periods and one time in five of the fast periods. In the frequency ratio 1:3, the same phase interrelation occurs in each slow period and in each third of the fast periods.

The influence from the former generator to the latter one may introduce a rhythmic reset in the second generator, where the number of such resets per time unit and the maximum time displacement per interaction decide the maximum frequency drive. For example, if a maximum displacement of 10 msec occurs, the resulting drive or frequency modulation of the driven generator is expected to be ±5% in the ratio 1:2, ±3.3% in the ratio 1:3 and only ±2% in the ratio 1:2.5. When the high frequency dominates, the harmonic interrelations are most pronounced in the ratio 1:3, but the ratio 1:2.5

is more represented when the high- and low-frequency components are nearly equal. These findings may indicate that an independent alpha frequency and independent low-frequency rhythm on an average have a frequency ratio between 1:2.5 and 1:3 or that a large-amplitude alpha is able to catch the low-frequency generator to a higher extent than a small-amplitude alpha and that the driving in the 1:2.5 ratio occurs in spite of the low driving possibilities ($\pm2\%$ per 10 msec), possibly because the uninfluenced frequency ratio as an average is closer to the 1:2.5 than to the 1:3 ratio.

(2) *The alpha waves produce events, the repetition periods of which are alternating multiples of the alpha period.* The low-frequency activity is considered as superposed events or transients being triggered by the alpha waves, with repetition periods being multiples of the alpha wave duration. An "event generator" may be released by for instance each alpha wave (1:1), every second alpha wave (1:2) and every third alpha wave (1:3). In this connection, the 2.5 relation may occur if the single generators are released alternatively by every second and every third alpha wave. The dominance of 4 Hz activity in the present material may, according to this explanation indicate a most probable relative latency time of approximately two alpha periods. Assuming that the latency periods which follow two stimuli are shorter the longer the interstimuli interval and assuming a latency period of approximately two alpha periods, an alternation between intervals of two and three alpha periods may persist in the reaction pattern to the stimulation originating in alpha generators. If the latency time is constantly less than two alpha periods, activity in the ratio 1:2 will appear; on the contrary, activity in the ratio 1:3 will be the result if the latency time is constantly slightly greater than two periods.

It is difficult to judge whether the two frequencies are generated due to interaction between two generators as proposed in explanation 1 or whether both frequencies, as in explanation 2, are generated by interaction between equal elements in a common generator structure. Explanation 2 may, however, be difficult to accept on the basis of the striking regularity in the wave form repetition which often characterizes slow posterior EEG rhythm. A further investigation by means of cross-reverse correlation may be helpful in exploring this problem.

SUMMARY

Slow posterior rhythmic activity in the frequency range 2.5–4.5 Hz was recorded from 40 adult patients and analyzed with the aid of a reverse correlator. The material shows strong rhythmic interdependence between the alpha wave frequency and the frequency of the slow rhythmic waves. The rhythmic interdependence was most pronounced in the frequency ratio 1:3, and, unexpectedly, in the 1:2.5 ratio. A lower interdependence was found in the 1:2 ratio. Two models for the simultaneous generation of activity in fixed-frequency interrelation are suggested.

ACKNOWLEDGMENT

This investigation was supported by grants from the Swedish Council of Applied Research, the Swedish Medical Research Council and the University of Göteborg, Sweden.

REFERENCES

Aird, R. B., and Gastaut, Y. (1959): Occipital and posterior electroencephalographic rhythm. *Electroencephalography and Clinical Neurophysiology*, II:637–656.

Eeg-Olofsson, O. (1970): The development of the EEG in normal children and adolescents. *Acta Paediatrica Scandinavica*, Suppl. 208.

Hambert, O., and Petersén, I. (1970): Clinical, electroencephalographical and neuropharmacological studies in syndromes of progressive myoclonus epilepsy. *Acta Neurologica Scandinavica*, 46:149–186.

Kaiser, E., Magnusson, R., and Petersén, I. (1967): Reverse correlation: a narrow-window autocorrelation technique for continuous analysis of frequency interrelations in non-stationary time series. *Digest of the 7th International Conference on Medicine and Biology*, p. 261.

Kaiser, E., and Petersén, I. (1965): A new method for detecting rhythmic activity in time series. In: *Communications, 6th International Congress of Electroencephalography and Clinical Neurophysiology*, Vienna, pp. 535–537.

Kaiser, E., and Petersén, I. (1968): Automatic analysis in EEG. I. Tapecomputer system for spectral analysis. II. Reverse correlation. *Acta Neurologica Scandinavica*, Suppl. 22:5–38.

Kaiser, E., and Petersén, I. (1968): Reverse correlation of 14 and 6 per second positive spikes. In: *Clinical Electroencephalography of Children*, edited by P. Kellaway and I. Petersén. Almqvist & Wiksell, Stockholm, pp. 155–166.

Kuhlo, W. (1967): Die 4–5/sec EEG-Grundrhythmusvariante im Schlaf und nach Contusio cerebri. *Archiv für Psychiatrie und Nervenkrankheiten*, 210:68–75.

Kuhlo, W., Heintel, H., and Vogel, F. (1969): The 4–5 c/sec rhythm. *Electroencephalography and Clinical Neurophysiology*, 26:613–618.

Nayrac, P., and Beaussart, M. (1956): A propos des rythmes à 4 c/s chez les anciens traumatisés craniens. *Revue Neurologique*, 94:189–191.

Petersén, I., Hambert, O., Kaiser, E., Magnusson, R., and Sörbye, R. (1969): Slow posterior EEG rhythms in syndromes of progressive myoclonus epilepsy. *Electroencephalography and Clinical Neurophysiology*, 26:340.

Petersén, I., and Sörbye, R. (1962): Slow posterior rhythm in adults. *Electroencephalography and Clinical Neurophysiology*, 14:161–170.

Pitot, M., and Gastaut, Y. (1956): Aspects électroencéphalographiques inhibituels des séquelles des traumatismes craniens: Les rythmes postérieurs à 4 cycles-seconde. *Revue Neurologique*, 94:189–191.

Selldén, U. (1964): Electroencephalographic activation with megimide in normal subjects. *Acta Neurologica Scandinavica*, 40 (Suppl. 12):30.

Vallat, J. N., and Lepetit, J. M. (1957): Presentation de tracés de traumatismes craniens avec rythmes postérieurs à quatre cycles-seconde. Notions sur les caractères évolutifs. Quelques réflexions à propos de l'experties. *Revue Neurologique*, 96:551–552.

Vogel, F., and Götze, W. (1959): Familienuntersuchungen zur Genetik des normalen Elektro-encephalogramms. *Deutsche Zeitschrift für Nervenheilkunde*, 178:668–700.

Automation of Clinical Electroencephalography.
Edited by P. Kellaway and I. Petersén.
Raven Press, New York © 1973.

The Detection and Quantification of Transient and Paroxysmal EEG Abnormalities

J. R. G. Carrie

Department of Neurophysiology, The Methodist Hospital, and Baylor College of Medicine, Houston, Texas 77025

If one asks an electroencephalographer why he considers that a particular segment of EEG shows an abnormal pattern, he will usually reply to the effect that it differs from the surrounding background activity. Thus, in the context of the electroencephalographer's perception of an "episodic," "transient" or "paroxysmal" abnormality, the features of the waveform found within the abnormal segment of the EEG cannot be specified in absolute terms but can be defined only in relation to the overall characteristics of the signal from which the transient abnormality arises. For example, a waveform that would be considered abnormally sharp in one record might not be rated as abnormal in another tracing in which the signal included a relatively greater amount of high frequency activity in the background. These concepts are implied in the definitions of "transient" and "paroxysm," proposed by the I.F.E.C.N. Terminology Committee (Storm van Leeuwen Chairman, 1966). Therefore, any technique that is in any way concerned with simulating the process of human identification of EEG episodic transient abnormalities must estimate the characteristics of the background activity and then relate measurements from each consecutive wave or group of waves to this estimate.

An electroencephalographer is often vague about defining the precise difference between a paroxysmal and abnormal pattern and the background activity from which it arises, but the greater the degree of confidence with which he can identify waves that are relatively sharper than the background waveforms, the more readily will he diagnose potentially epileptogenic dysfunction. This clinical diagnostic confidence in relation to waveforms that appear to be sharply contoured at the most commonly used recording speeds is justified by numerous published electro-clinical correlative studies. This chapter is therefore concerned mainly with discussing the problems involved in detecting and quantifying EEG patterns that include what the human electroencephalographer perceives as sharp transients, although the technique that is described could be adapted for use in detecting paroxysmal EEG abnormalities of any kind.

To develop a system for the automatic detection of EEG waveforms that are sharper than other waves in the signal, it is first necessary to specify the types of waveform measurement which are to be tested as indicators of sharpness.

Visual inspection of EEG spikes and sharp waves suggests that they differ from background activity in that they exhibit rapid rising and falling phases. Therefore, one may predict that a sharp transient would show a relatively high maximal value of the first derivative of the EEG signal with respect to time when compared with the background EEG activity. However, the appearance of sharpness on visual inspection refers mainly to the contour seen at the peaks or troughs of a waveform. In a spike or sharp wave, the first derivative of the voltage signal with respect to time changes relatively rapidly at the peak or trough of the wave. One would therefore expect that the most sensitive measurement of sharpness in a waveform would be the rate of rate of voltage change, *i.e.*, the second derivative of the signal with respect to time.

In the light of the foregoing considerations, the work discussed here was designed: (1) to develop a technique to determine the extent to which abnormal EEG transients differ from the average of the surrounding background activity in terms of specific waveform measurements; (2) to determine which waveform measurements detect abnormal transients most efficiently, with special reference to the first and second derivatives of the signal with respect to time; and (3) to explore the possibility of using the above findings as a basis for developing a recognition system for detecting and quantifying abnormal EEG patterns such as spike-and-wave discharges while excluding artifacts.

METHOD

The transient detection and analysis system that has been developed can be used either online or offline using a signal that has been recorded previously on magnetic tape. The amplified signal is transmitted through lines to the computer room and is then either entered directly to the input of a digital computer (LINC-8 or PDP-12) or is first processed by an analog computer. The analog computer is programmed either as a differentiator or as a two-stage successive differentiator to provide the first or second derivative of the EEG signal with respect to time. The high frequencies of the signal are attenuated by analog filters to reduce unwanted noise when either the first or second derivative is used as the input to the digital computer.

Figure 1 illustrates the general features of the digital program. In its present form, the system can process information from only one EEG channel. The digital program causes the computer to compare consecutive measurements in the EEG signal, or a derived function of this signal, with a moving average of similar measurements from a pre-set number of preceding waves. In the work described here, the voltage levels at the peaks and troughs of the waves were measured for each wave. The number of waves contributing to the average is determined by sense switch settings at the time the program is loaded into the computer memory and consists of a maximum of 256 waves. At the end of each wave, a check is made to see whether the magnitude of the measurement from the latest wave exceeds the average of measurements from the preceding waves by a pre-set threshold ratio. If the threshold is not exceeded, the moving average is updated, and the sampling of information from the next wave proceeds immediately. If the threshold is exceeded, an abnormality indication or evaluation sequence is initiated.

At the simplest level, the program causes generation of a pulse that puts an indicator mark on the graphic EEG recording to draw attention to the occurrence of a quantitatively unusual wave. This, of course, leaves most of the evaluation work to the human electroencephalographer. At the opposite end of the scale, the computer does all the pattern recognition and evaluation work automatically, either rejecting the information as artifact or nonpathological or, on the other hand, rating it as abnormal and storing the information for inclusion in some kind of output display at the end of the analysis period. At the present time, the system transfers all the spatial analysis problems to the human electroencephalographer. However the system can be programmed to detect and to analyze automatically EEG abnormalities occurring in one channel where the properties of the abnormal segment in the time (or frequency) domain are clearly distinguished from those of the preceding background signal. These properties are perceived by the human electroencephalographer as the "morphology" of the EEG signal. When adjusted to look for spike-and-wave, the system detects the occurrence of an abnormal pattern when waves of a specified degree of sharpness in relation to the preceding background activity are closely as-

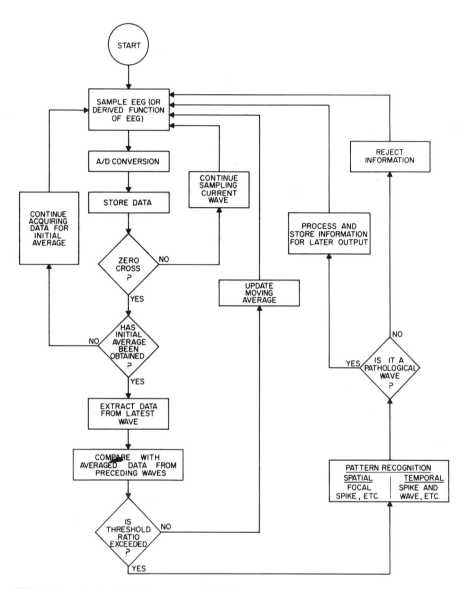

FIG. 1. Flow chart of digital program for EEG transient detection and analysis.

sociated with slow waves of specified duration. At the end of each abnormal segment of EEG, the information about the occurrence of EEG abnormalities is brought up to date and stored for output at the end of the analysis period. The most recent version of the system, which uses a PDP-12 computer, provides a quantitative output showing the number of abnormal paroxysms and their average duration.

The digital program is started, stopped, and reinitialized by pushing a button on the EEG recorder console, and a console light switches on automatically while the program is running. The results of the analysis are printed out as hard copy on a Teletype teletypewriter and are also displayed in the recording room on the screen of a CRT display terminal.

RESULTS

Comparison of First and Second Derivative Analysis

The technique described above can be used to identify the waveform measurements that discriminate most efficiently between specified types of abnormal paroxysmal waves and background activity in an EEG signal (Carrie, 1972). It has been found that the second derivative with respect to time is a more efficient discriminator of sharp transients than the first derivative. In some situations the discriminatory efficiency of the two derivatives is closely similar; however, the first derivative reaches a relatively high value in response to the high rate of voltage change that occurs in waves of large amplitude which are not necessarily sharply contoured. Thus, in some EEG samples containing small-amplitude spikes and large-amplitude slow waves, the highest value for the second derivative occurred during the spikes, but the maximal value for the first derivative was developed during the slow waves.

Detection of Paroxysmal EEG Patterns

The upper tracing in Fig. 2 shows a segment of EEG signal that includes a burst of spike-and-wave activity. The second tracing shows the selective amplification of the spikes in the filtered second derivative of the EEG signal with respect to time. The third tracing shows the output from the digital computer programmed to generate a rectangular pulse when a wave occurred in the second derivative whose amplitude was three or more times greater than a moving average of the amplitude of the preceding 256 waves in that channel; *i.e.*, a pulse was generated when a wave in the EEG signal was three or more times sharper than the average sharpness of the preceding

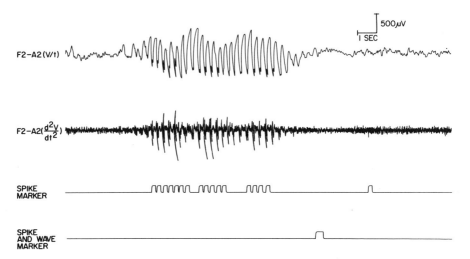

FIG. 2. Channel 1: EEG signal that includes burst of spike-and-wave. Channel 2: Filtered second derivative of the EEG signal with respect to time, showing selective amplification of sharply contoured waves. Channel 3: Output from digital computer marking the occurrence of waves three or more times as sharp as the average sharpness of the preceding 256 waves. Channel 4: Output from digital computer marking the end of the preceding burst of spike and wave, when the computer was programmed to respond specifically to spike-and-wave patterns. There is one pulse at the end of the burst of spike-and-wave, but the sharp transient occurring approximately 3 sec later is not rated abnormal.

waves. There are 16 pulses during the burst of spike-and-wave, and a single isolated pulse approximately 3 sec after the end of the burst at the time of a small-amplitude, sharply contoured wave in the EEG signal. The lowest channel shows the output from the digital computer when it was programmed to detect waves that were three or more times sharper than the waves in the preceding background signal and which were closely associated with slow waves of specified duration. Having detected the sharp transients associated with slow waves during the paroxysmal discharge, the computer waits until the burst of abnormal activity has ended before a marker pulse is generated; it ignores the isolated sharp transient occurring 3 sec after the burst. Many minutes of tape recorded signals have been analyzed by the spike-and-wave detection system. These records included "sharp" switch artifacts, montage changes, and muscle potentials, but the spike-and-wave detector indicated an abnormal pattern only when a spike-and-wave pattern occurred which met the specified quantitative criteria.

DISCUSSION OF RESULTS

A small number of techniques for the identification of specific EEG patterns have been described in the literature. Kaiser and Petersén (1968) described a device that uses reverse correlation for identifying 14 and 6/sec positive spikes. Bickford (1959) described a system that detected waveforms of a specified frequency whose amplitude exceeded a preset threshold; this system was useful in the electrographic and clinical investigation of patients suffering from petit mal epilepsy who showed a 3/sec spike-and-wave EEG pattern. The technique described in this report has been applied so far to the detection and quantification of spike-and-wave in the EEG. This, however, represents a specific application of a more general approach to the problem of detecting transient and paroxysmal abnormalities. The system developed in the present investigation does not look for waves meeting certain fixed criteria in terms of amplitude and duration, as in the technique developed by Bickford; instead, the background activity is examined, and the threshold (microvolt level or millisecond duration) for activating the spike-and-wave detection sequence is adapted to the average characteristics of the EEG signal that is being generated.

The initial part of the present investigation was concerned with developing a technique that would identify waves whose sharpness exceeded that of the background activity by a predetermined specification. The voltage levels at the peaks and troughs of the second derivative of the EEG signal were found to be the most suitable measurements for this purpose. However, in determining whether a particular transient pattern is or is not pathological and in determining whether it is or is not an artifact, the human electroencephalographer uses information such as events at adjacent electrodes and the presence or absence of abnormally slow elements following the sharply contoured wave in addition to the quality of sharpness. In this study, the response specificity of the system has been increased by programming, which causes it to indicate the occurrence of an abnormality only when it detects a spike-and-wave pattern — an abnormally sharp waveform (in relation to the background EEG) together with a following wave or waves of specified slowness. Two main lines of further development are being followed. Firstly, the system described in this investigation is being modified so that the spike and wave detector uses additional information from the EEG signal and extracts the information from several channels. Secondly, construction of a device using analog hardware that will perform some of the digital operations carried out in the present hybrid system is under consideration. Such a device would simplify the process of automatically detecting and quantifying some EEG patterns and would reduce the cost involved. In addition to these two main lines of development, a preliminary study is being made of the application of this approach to the detection and localization of focal transient abnormalities.

The technique described in this chapter is a prototype of a system that will utilize standardized criteria to provide consistency in the evaluation and quantification of EEG transient and paroxysmal abnormalities. It will also reduce the time spent by skilled personnel in data interpretation and measurement. However, this method can at best equal or slightly improve on the performance of the human electroencephalographer in regard to the detection and evaluation of individual transients. It is possible that the application of more complex techniques may result in the development of EEG transient detectors which are more sensitive than the human visual analyzer. Some aspects of these techniques are discussed by other authors elsewhere in this volume.

The conceptual approach used in developing the present system applies to the detection of episodic, transient or paroxysmal abnormalities. In a small proportion of subjects who suffer from seizures, the EEG is continuously abnormal and sharply contoured waves represent a considerable proportion of all the waves that are present. This situation is seen, for example, in some patients with hypsarrhythmic EEGs. In this instance, where many sharp transients are present, the electroencephalographer probably does not define sharpness in relation to an estimate of the average sharpness of the waves in the record that he is examining; instead, he recognizes that nonperiodic waves are present which occur frequently and exceed in sharpness the majority of the waves that he has seen in other records. He therefore switches to a different perceptual program that uses an arbitrary standard of sharpness based on stored information from previous experience. The system described in this paper, whose "experience" is, at most, 256 waves long, could not cope with these types of records, but appropriate modification and extension should not be unduly difficult.

SUMMARY

A technique is described which detects transient abnormalities in an EEG signal by comparing measurements from consecutive waves in the signal with a moving average of similar measurements from the preceding waves. The evidence up to the present time suggests that the second derivative of the signal with respect to time provides the measurements that discriminate sharp transients most efficiently. A system is described which responds specifically to spike-and-wave paroxysmal discharges and quantifies this type of abnormal activity. General aspects of the problem of detecting and quantifying EEG transient and paroxysmal abnormalities are discussed.

DISCUSSION

Magnusson asked whether the amplitude detector had been applied to the raw EEG as well as to the undifferentiated signal. Carrie replied that this had not been done, since measurements of wave amplitude do not of themselves provide information about the sharpness of a wave. In the spike-and-wave discriminator, wave duration but not wave amplitude information was extracted from the undifferentiated EEG signal as part of the process of abnormality detection. In some circumstances, however, detection of wave amplitude, or of relative wave amplitude with respect to the amplitude of background activity, might be useful in discriminating certain types of paroxysmal abnormality.

Saltzberg said that his group had employed measurements of the second derivative in detecting EEG spikes in schizophrenic research several years ago. They had found that waves which a human electroencephalographer selected as being abnormally sharp were approximately three times as sharp on the second derivative criterion as sharply contoured waves in the background which were not rated visually as abnormal. Saltzberg agreed with Frost, who suggested that a simple system of this type would necessarily detect sharply contoured artifact as well as spikes due to intracerebral pathology. Carrie commented that a human electroencephalographer uses a considerable amount of information other than that relating to wave sharpness in differentiating pathological patterns which include sharply contoured waves from those due to noncerebral biological potentials such as muscle or nonbiological artifact. Consequently, in developing a technique that could discriminate a particular type of abnormal EEG pattern, i.e., spike-and-wave, it had been necessary to develop a system which evaluates quantitatively several aspects of the EEG signal and which adjusts the threshold for initiating the abnormality detection sequence according to the average characteristics of the preceding background activity.

Kaiser said that he would have expected that successive differentiation of the EEG would result in so much selective amplification of the noise in the signal that analysis would be virtually impossible. Carrie agreed that this was a problem. It had been tackled in two ways. (1) The signal was subjected to analog filtering before and after successive differentiation, resulting in substantial attenuation of components between 30 and 100 Hz, with marked attenuation above 100 Hz. (2) The digital program could be easily adjusted to reject waves of less than the specified duration. This had proved useful in eliminating the effects of spurious zero crossings due to noise that might occur shortly before and soon after the zero crossings of the true signal.

Dumermuth asked if the system could discriminate spikes within a signal containing a large amount of fast activity. Carrie replied that the EEG patterns which are discriminated out of the background by a system of this type depend on the parameters that one inserts into the program. If one uses the same parameters that a human uses for detection purposes, the system will detect the same patterns. The situation mentioned by the questioner was a specific example of the more general problem of discriminating specific abnormal events where the quantitative characteristics of the abnormal waves differed by less than usual from those of the background waves. In these circumstances, the detector will not discriminate better than the human but will perform as efficiently. Thus, where the human sees a pattern that he cannot rate with certainty as pathological or nonpathological, such as a sharply contoured wave that arises in a background containing much fast activity, an automatic system of this type will also be unreliable in regard to its discriminatory performance. However, the computer system will give perfect test-retest reliability since it always uses the same quantitatively definable criteria.

REFERENCES

Bickford, R. G. (1959): An automatic recognition system for spike-and-wave with simultaneous testing of motor response. *Electroencephalography and Clinical Neurophysiology,* 11:397–398.

Carrie, J. R. G. (1972): A technique for analyzing EEG transient abnormalities. *Electroencephalography and Clinical Neurophysiology,* 32:199–201.

Kaiser, E., and Petersén, I. (1968): Reverse correlation of 14 and 6 per second positive spikes. In: *Clinical Electroencephalography of Children,* edited by P. Kellaway and I. Petersén. Almqvist & Wiksell, Stockholm, pp. 155–166.

Storm van Leeuwen, W. (Chairman), Bickford, R., Brazier, M., Cobb, W. A., Dondey, H., Gastaut, H., Gloor, P., Henry, C. E., Hess, R., Knott, J. R., Kugler, J., Lairy, G. C., Loeb, C., Magnus, O., Oller Daurella, L., Petsche, N., Schwab, R., Walter, W. G., and Widén, L. (1966): Proposal for EEG terminology by the terminology committee of the International Federation for Electroencephalography and Clinical Neurophysiology. *Electroencephalography and Clinical Neurophysiology,* 20:306–310.

Automation of Clinical Electroencephalography.
Edited by P. Kellaway and I. Petersén.
Raven Press, New York © 1973.

Spike Detection by Computer and by Analog Equipment

Lars H. Zetterberg

Royal Institute of Technology, Electrical Engineering Department, Telecommunication Theory, Stockholm 70, Sweden

SPIKE DETECTION BY MEANS OF COMPUTER

A preceding report (Zetterberg, *this volume*), discusses EEG signals that appear to be realizations of a stationary stochastic process when recorded for approximately 20 sec. However, it is well known that not all registrations may be classified as such. We notice drastic changes in the EEG signal when the eyes are opened or closed, and muscle activities give rise to specific pulses or transients which are easy to detect by the experienced clinician. Another form of pulses called spikes or sharp waves appear in recordings from patients who have a form of brain injury called cortical epilepsy. These spikes occur together with the normal EEG activity, and it is of considerable clinical interest to detect the presence of these pulses. When the present work was started, the goal was to achieve at least as good results as a clinician may do and possibly better. This seems to be a reasonable expectation, considering the efficiency of known methods for pulse detection by means of matched filters. Notice, however, that the noise here is the normal EEG activity which may be described as colored rather than white noise.

A closer look at the situation reveals the following facts. Certain spikes stand out quite clearly against the background, as the two upper curves in Fig. 1. However, in many cases the pulses are strongly disturbed by the normal EEG activity. We have worked on the hypothesis that for one in-

227

dividual the pulse form is about the same for various spikes but the amplitude may vary. As seen in Fig. 1, spikes appear simultaneously in two channels, a fact that has been taken advantage of by employing a coincidence logic. It should be noted that the pulse forms for two such channels may not be quite the same due to the different location of the electrode pairs relative to the epileptic focus. This may lead to a differentiation of the primary pulse (Herolf, 1971). Also, the pulses may not occur quite coincidentally.

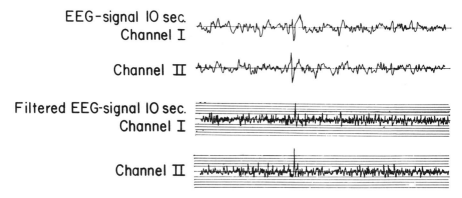

FIG. 1. Example of spike detection by computer.

What is the pulse form of a spike? In Fig. 2, a pulse is shown for one individual, or rather the average pulse form found by taking the sum of several large spikes. Approximately the same pulse shape will appear with other individuals, but the time scale for the mean pulse may differ from that of the figure. It has been observed that the later parts of the pulses for one individual may vary from one occasion to another, although they are fairly

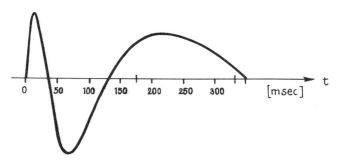

FIG. 2. Example of average pulse form for one individual.

stable during the first 0.2 sec. This conclusion is used to represent the pulse as a vector $\bar{p}$ with 20 components assuming a sampling rate of 100 Hz.

$$\bar{p} = (p_0, p_1, \ldots, p_m)$$

The general theory for detecting a pulse in noise says that the received signal should be put through a suitable filter, and the decision should be based on the output of the filter. If the output exceeds in absolute value a certain threshold, the presence of a pulse is announced. In order to formulate the algorithm, it seems reasonable to assume that the pulse is added to the normal EEG activity. The filter is described by the following vector $\bar{c} = (c_0, c_1, \ldots, c_m)$ and the filter operation by the relation

$$y_t = c_0 x_t + c_1 x_{t-1} + \ldots + c_m x_{t-m}$$

where x_t is the sampled EEG signal. The filter is specified by maximizing the signal-to-noise ratio

$$\frac{||\bar{c}^T \bar{p}||}{\bar{c}^T R \bar{c}}$$

with respect to $\bar{c}$. $R = (r_{i-j})$ is the covariance matrix of the background activity which is closely approximated by the covariance matrix of the received EEG signal. The optimal filter vector may be put in closed form

$$\bar{c}_{\text{opt}} = R^{-1} \bar{p}$$

The present procedure (Herolf, 1971) for detecting spikes by making use of a computer follows. The pulse form is supposed to be known.

1. Select an appropriate interval.
2. Employ A/D-conversion with 100 samples/sec and divide observation time in sections of 10-sec length.
3. Compute the autocovariance coefficients $\{r_k\}$ and also $\bar{c}_{\text{opt}}$.
4. Perform digital filtering of one or two channels.
5. Classify the output signal in various amplitude intervals, and combine the information for two channels.
6. Plot the original and filtered signal with threshold levels.

Figure 1 contains an example where the two lower curves depict the filtered signals. Table 1 summarizes the results of an analysis of 240 sec of recording. The number of samples in different amplitude levels is shown for channels 1 and 2 and also the combined information for both channels. In this example we have required, in order to accept coincidence, that the two pulses will have the amplitudes in the same range. Evidently the coincidence logic reduces the number of small-amplitude pulses while it accepts only

TABLE 1. Result of analysis of 240 sec of registration on two channels

Absolute signal level	Channel I	Channel II	Channel I & II
$3 - 4\sigma$	35	24	1
$4 - 5\sigma$	9	9	1
$5 - 6\sigma$	10	2	0
$> 6\sigma$	18	25	16

σ^2 = signal variance.

moderately the strong ones. Notice that they have an amplitude larger than 6σ where σ is the standard deviation. The probability of a false indication is here negligible, a result that also checks with visual inspection. For further details, see Herolf (1971), which also includes results for other coincidence criteria.

Another example of spike detection is given in Fig. 3. In the upper two traces, channel A and B, the spikes are clearly visible in channel A but much less so in channel B. Only the information in channel B has been used for spike detection, and the result is shown in the last two traces. The upper curve is once more channel B, but with a different time scale and with sign reversal; the last curve shows the filtered output. Again the spikes stand out quite clearly.

These examples show promising results, but a clinical evaluation of the

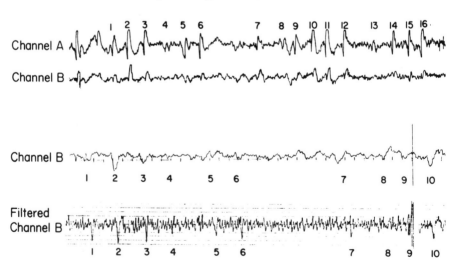

FIG. 3. Example of spike detection by computer.

method has not yet been carried out. Actually a member of our group, M. Herolf, is working on an improved version of the algorithm where the pulse form need not be measured in advance.

SPIKE DETECTION BY MEANS OF ANALOG EQUIPMENT

The block diagram of the spike detector is reproduced in Fig. 4. It contains detectors for two channels and logic that will combine this information in various ways. Each channel contains an amplifier and two filters that will essentially whiten the spectrum of the normal EEG activity. The first of these filters suppresses the δ-activity, whereas the second one suppresses

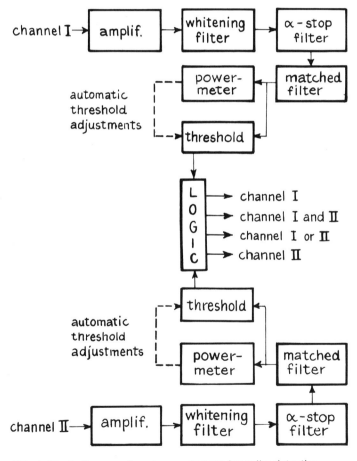

FIG. 4. Block diagram of analog equipment for spike detection.

the α-activity. They are designed as first- and second-order active RC filters, respectively. With these precautions, the detector filter may be constructed to match the pulse form as it appears after the whitening filters. Two threshold levels, one for positive and one for negative values, are adjusted automatically by measuring also the RMS value or actually the mean of the rectified EEG signal using a suitable integration constant. The logic takes into account a small possible difference in time of arrival for pulses from the two channels.

Figure 5 gives an example of spike detection where we can see the original signal for channel I and II and the results after they have been filtered. The last line contains the output from the logic requiring coincidence of pulses. Clearly the two spikes are detected, and no false pulses are indicated.

A test was run on a 3-min EEG recording where the clinician had information available from all 16 channels recorded. When a comparison was made, we found that a threshold setting of Tr6 (3.4σ) gave 15 spike indications out of the 17 given by the clinician, and moreover, one indication that was classified as a possible spike. With a lower threshold setting, there is a definite risk for false indications. To see this, we have shown in Fig. 6 the operating characteristic curves for each channel and for the combined ones. Each diagram contains one curve that shows the number of actual spike

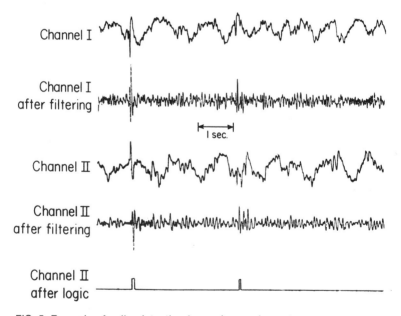

FIG. 5. Example of spike detection by analog equipment.

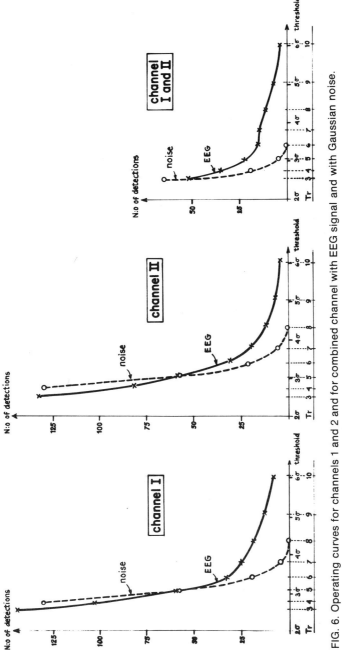

FIG. 6. Operating curves for channels 1 and 2 and for combined channel with EEG signal and with Gaussian noise.

indications for the 3 min sequence and also the expected number of indications that would result if the EEG signal was a Gaussian process with the same RMS value as has been measured. Clearly the number of actual spike indications is much larger than we expect with pure noise when the threshold is Tr6 or above. The combined channel reduces the number of false indications considerably.

The equipment is presently being used at the Karolinska Hospital for testing purposes. It was constructed by L.-Å. Dahlman.

DISCUSSION

Walter asked if the bleaching filters had to be carefully adjusted to permit satisfactory operation of the detector. Zetterberg replied that on the basis of experience to date, this adjustment did not appear to be critical. However, a more definite answer could be given to this question when some recordings of long duration in practical situations had been obtained. Zetterberg accepted Kaiser's comment that since the matched filter used a window of 200 msec, there would be some interaction between spikes with an interspike interval shorter than 200 msec.

REFERENCES

Herolf, M. (1971): Detection of pulse-shaped signals in EEG. *Technical Report No. 41, Telecommunication Theory*. Royal Institute of Technology, Stockholm.

Automation of Clinical Electroencephalography.
Edited by P. Kellaway and I. Petersén.
Raven Press, New York © 1973.

A Method in Automatic Pattern Recognition in EEG

E. Kaiser, I. Petersén and R. Magnusson

Kaiser Laboratory, Copenhagen, Denmark, Department of Clinical Neurophysiology, Sahlgren Hospital, Göteborg, and Department of Applied Electronics, Chalmer's University of Technology, Göteborg, Sweden

After the early papers of Grass and Gibbs (1938), Drohocki (1939), and Drohocki and Drohocka (1939) concerning Fourier analysis and recording of amplitude spectra, the first decade of automatic analysis of EEG was concentrated on analysis in the frequency and amplitude domain.

The next step into operation on the time-amplitude pattern was taken by Dawson (1947, 1954) with the introduction of the superposition method and, later on, automatic time averaging of stimulus-related activity.

The availability of digital computers and algorithms for efficient use of automatic data processing has especially favored the use of spectral information and time averaging in expressing EEG patterns, whereas the less complex wave patterns in spontaneous activity are still evaluated by visual examination.

Various approaches have been taken to detect events of different kinds by automatic methods.

Conventional approaches for detection of specific events include analog or digital filtering to isolate or at least to improve the signal-to-noise ratio before the wanted signal is passed into a level detector.

A more universal solution was proposed by Kaiser and Sem-Jacobsen (1962) and Sem-Jacobsen and Kaiser (1964), who introduced a plurality of threshold levels in the time-and-amplitude domain. In this way each consecutive EEG wave was represented by eight bits expressing amplitude-and-frequency class.

An important step in simplification and avoidance of redundant information in the EEG was taken by Cohn, Leader, Weiker and Caceres (1967). The digital EEG signal was preprocessed and represented in the computer memory by the coordinates in time and voltage of its amplitude peaks including significant secondary wave minima.

A multichannel-wave pattern digitizer intended to serve as a signal conditioner for subsequent computer evaluation was described by Kaiser, Petersén and Magnusson (1970).

Each consecutive EEG full-wave was expressed in a 14-bit data-word covering the frequency, the duty, the amplitude class, the number of secondary waves, and the presence and polarity of possible spikes.

METHOD

After appropriate LF filtering, 16 EEG signals are passed into an A/D converter via a sample-and-hold multiplexer working at a sampling frequency of 200 Hz in each channel. Block diagrams of the system are shown in Figs. 1 and 2. The digital output is stored in a core memory enabling 16-channel epoch storage of approximately 4 sec. At the end of each storage period, a fast processing of the stored information takes place without disturbing the running sampling and storage of new input data (Fig. 3). The processing takes place at a speed which is 133 times the data-input speed.

Operations on the time pattern of each consecutive full-wave is based on the time of zero-crossings.

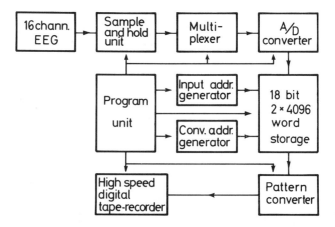

FIG. 1. General block diagram of the processing arrangement.

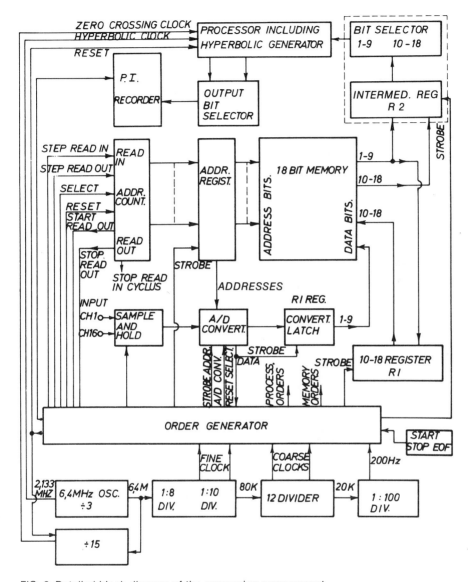

FIG. 2. Detailed block diagram of the processing arrangement.

As the sampling frequency is only 200 Hz, an intermediate 16-point interpolation routine is introduced in order to increase the accuracy. By means of a hyperbolic generator, the duration of each full-wave is converted to equivalent frequency. The frequency is classed in steps of 1 Hz in the

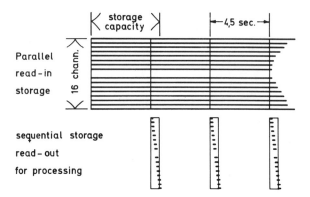

FIG. 3. Timing diagram. Sixteen-channel sequential information is fed to the memory at a constant sampling rate. When $7/8$ of the memory addresses are loaded, a fast read-out and processing sequence is initiated. The read-in (write) is maintained undisturbed during this procedure. The processing is performed at a rate which is 133 times the read-in velocity.

range of 1 to 31 Hz (five bits). Two bits more are used to express the time pattern; the first bit indicates if the first half-wave has a duration of less than half the duration of the second half-wave (positive duty; Fig. $4G_2$), and the next bit indicates if the first half-wave has a duration of more than twice that of the second half-wave (negative duty; Fig. $4G_1$). The amplitude pattern is expressed via the class of the peak-to-peak amplitude expressed in eight classes having the amplitude ratio 1:2:4:8 and so on.

Three bits are used to indicate the amplitude class. The number of secondary half-waves is indicated by two bits expressing the presence of zero, one, two, or more than two secondary waves. The presence of secondary waves are indicated if secondary minima in the full-wave shows deviation from the amplitude peak of more than 25% of the full-wave amplitude (Fig. 4C, D, E).

The presence and polarity of spikes are processed in a filter-like digital operation based on summation of the first and second derivative.

The sensitivity threshold is arbitrarily set to be met by a 50-Hz signal having a peak-to-peak amplitude of 50 μV.

A new routine is introduced in order to cope with difficulties when, for example, slow waves and alpha activity are present at nearly the same amplitude. Three routines are introduced in order to deal with adjacent waves.

Routine I (Fig. 4B): If the amplitude of the second half-wave is less than 25% of the previous half-wave, the next full-wave is included in the total duration, and the first wave is indicated as only a secondary wave.

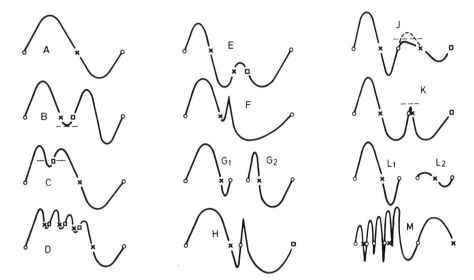

FIG. 4. Demonstration of processing properties.

A: Normal wave characterized solely by duration-to-frequency conversion and peak-to-peak amplitude class. B: The termination of the first full-wave is neglected because its second half-wave is below 25% of the peak-to-peak value. Only one full-wave is accepted plus one secondary wave (Routine I). C: One secondary wave is detected because the intermediate minimum deviates from the preceding peak more than 25% of the peak-to-peak value. D: More than two secondary waves are detected. E: One secondary wave is detected. F: Detection is like that in B. G_1: Negative duty is indicated. G_2: Positive duty is indicated. H: Two consecutive waves are interrelated because positive duty is preceded by negative duty. Subsequent treatment combines the two waves and indicates one secondary wave (Routine III). J: Two consecutive waves are interrelated because the first half-wave in the second full-wave is 25% below the peak-to-peak value (Routine II). K: Two consecutive waves to be treated like J. L_1: Normal wave like A. L_2: If L_2 follows L_1, its small size compared to L_1 causes same result as in J. M: Complicated wave pattern where the three first waves are detected as full-waves (spikes), and the following wave is detected as a wave at half the former frequencies having one secondary wave (spike).

Routine II (Fig. 4J, K): If the first half-wave has an amplitude less than 25% of the previous second half-wave, the two duty bits are used to indicate this situation in order to allow the subsequent processing to include the duration of the preceding full-wave and to indicate the last wave as a secondary wave.

This mentioned indication via the two duty bits is performed by indicating the contradictive statement that positive *and* negative duties are present in the full-wave.

In the case of a wave-and-spike pattern, the spike may divide one slow-wave into two full-waves of each half duration; this failure may be corrected in the final evaluation by routine III.

Routine III (Fig. 4H): If the duty of the first full-wave is negative and the duty of the second full-wave is positive in two consecutive waves, regard the two consecutive waves as one wave having twice the duration of the primary waves and add one secondary wave.

The final decision concerning a possible wave-and-spike pattern is later on a matter of the frequency and amplitude class and the spike detector information.

The output data appear sequentially in each channel, and the recording format allows subsequent investigation of simultaneous patterns in the different channels, their phase interrelations, and spatial patterns.

The converted data are not limited to the processing of sequential and spatial patterns. The information is also available for simple bookkeeping on the frequency-and-amplitude classes in order to obtain amplitude spectra and frequency-amplitude spectra.

DISCUSSION OF RESULTS

Detection based on comparisons between obtained sequences of full-wave words and stored-reference sequences should allow a reasonable tolerance concerning frequency class and amplitude class.

This tolerance may be performed by a referential presentation of a number of possible parameter combinations or by presenting the limits of the referential parameters.

In cases where the appearance of events is combined with minor shifts in the level of the background activity, a subsequent evaluation may take the advantage of the statistical nature of the EEG signal.

A current average of the amplitude classes improves the accuracy of the determination of the background level in spite of the coarse amplitude classing.

The period decision problems in connection with zero-crossing where complex signals are present have been dealt with by Burch (1959), who introduced the first and second derivative in order to obtain adequate information about secondary waves. The present treatment in the detection of secondary peaks and the use of information indicating adjacent waves as mentioned in the routines I, II and III are proposed as less sensitive to changes in frequency interrelations and better related to the visual appearance of the curves.

The goal of developing methods for automatic pattern recognition with resolution as good or better than the human eye is desirable but difficult to achieve.

SUMMARY

EEG patterns are expressed via the shape of sequential full-waves codified in a 14-bit data word. The parameters are frequency class, amplitude class, duty deviation, secondary waves, and the presence and polarity of spikes.

Logical operations are performed on complex interrelated adjacent waves on the basis of deviations in their time-and-amplitude pattern.

ACKNOWLEDGMENT

This investigation was supported in part by a grant from the Swedish Medical Research Council.

DISCUSSION

This report was followed by some discussion of the identification of the "secondary" waves, and some participants asked the speaker to describe the output of the detector in response to EEG wave patterns which they sketched on the blackboard. Saltzberg commented that detection of the zeroes of the first derivative waveform could provide some information about the secondary waves. For example, one could compute the total number of the secondary peaks from a simple count of derivative zero crossings. However, the inclusion of the 25% criterion used by the authors probably provides useful information in defining the characteristics of the EEG waveform.

REFERENCES

Burch, N. R. (1959): Automatic analysis of the electroencephalogram: a review and classification of systems. *Electroencephalography and Clinical Neurophysiology*, 11:827–834.

Cohn, R., Leader, H. S., Weiher, A. L., and Caceres, C. A. (1967): Computer mensuration and interpretation of the human EEG. *Digest of 7th International Conference on Medical and Biological Engineering*, Stockholm.

Dawson, G. D. (1947): Cerebral responses to electrical stimulation of peripheral nerves in man. *Journal of Neurology, Neurosurgery and Psychiatry*, 10:134–140.

Dawson, G. D. (1954): A summation technique for the detection of small evoked potentials. *Electroencephalography and Clinical Neurophysiology*, 6:65–84.

Drohocki, Z. (1939): Elektrospektographie des Gehirns. *Klinische Wochenschrift*, 18:536–538.

Drohocki, Z., and Drohocka, J. (1939): L'électrospectogramme du cerveau. *Comptes Rendus des Séances de la Société de Biologie et de ses Filiales*, 130:95–98.

Grass, A. M., and Gibbs, F. A. (1938): Fourier transform of the electroencephalogram. *Journal of Neurophysiology*, 1:521–526.

Kaiser, E., Petersén, I., and Magnusson, R. (1970): A sixteen-channel wave-pattern digitizer. *1st. Nordic Meeting on Medical and Biological Engineering*, Helsingfors, pp. 128–130.

Kaiser, E., and Sem-Jacobsen, C. W. (1962): "Yes-no" data reduction in EEG automatic pattern recognition. *Electroencephalography and Clinical Neurophysiology*, 14:955.

Sem-Jacobsen, C. W., and Kaiser, E. (1964): Collection of neurophysiological and cardiovascular data with data reduction, pattern and correlation analysis. *Symposium on the Analysis of Central Nervous System and Cardiovascular Data Using Computer Methods*. Washington, D.C., NASA SP-72.

Automation of Clinical Electroencephalography.
Edited by P. Kellaway and I. Petersén.
Raven Press, New York © 1973.

Classification and Discrimination of the EEG During Sleep

L. E. Larsen,* E. H. Ruspini, J. J. McNew, D. O. Walter, and W. R. Adey

Department of Anatomy and Space Biology Laboratory of the Brain Research Institute, University of California at Los Angeles, Los Angeles, California

I. INTRODUCTION

Sleep research, along with epilepsy, ranks among the most successful applications of electroencephalography in clinical neurophysiology. Indeed, the introduction of EEG made possible great strides in providing objective standards by which to stage sleep. This in turn stimulated interest in studies of electroclinical correlation with all its attendant problems of devising behavioral measures for depth of sleep. Although we are not attempting to minimize the importance of electroclinical correlation, whose solutions are central to the general brain/behavior problem, we shall limit our attention to the EEG as a product of the sleeping brain with only brief diversions into electroclinical correlations.

The emphasis of this volume is on the automation of clinical EEG analysis. It is axiomatic, therefore, than an automatic system for analysis of the EEG during sleep should emulate the end product, if not the process, of the clinical electroencephalographer. Within the area of sleep and coma, we would contend that the answer to this problem is well within reach, at least

---

*Division of Neuropsychiatry, Walter Reed Institute of Research, Walter Reed Army Medical Center, Washington, D.C.

in the case of longitudinal analysis. It is due, at least in part, to the results of emulating by machine the human sleep stage pattern-recognizing mechanism that a second generation of inquiry becomes of interest.

In order to expose the second generation question, it becomes necessary to consider the preceding results a little more closely. Most importantly, the first contribution of data analysis to sleep studies began with a pattern recognition problem; that is, given the classification system as prior information (most often, the Dement-Klietman sleep staging system as formalized by the APSS), the objective is to sort EEG epochs into one of the predetermined groups with minimal errors of allocation. Methods to meet this objective have had a substantial degree of success, as evidenced by preceding chapters in this volume. Yet it is by way of this very success, as well as certain clinical suspicions, that we are led to a second generation of inquiry: Is the present concept of sleep staging a good or even an adequate system to serve as prior information for sleep stage pattern recognition?

We note that the output of sleep staging machines shows much more variation than the output of the human pattern classifier. Indeed, it is common to all sleep stage recognition schemes that it is necessary to smooth the machines' output in order to arrive at decent agreement with the clinician. If we examine the epochs of disagreement, one finds that the clinical electroencephalographer makes his judgment as much by context as by the particular record. Often the record taken by itself is not clearly related to any of the categories provided by the classification system. Classification of such epochs is possible largely because there were epochs in the vicinity that were more clearly related to the classification system. It is on the basis of these selected epochs that a whole patch of EEG was classified. In fact, most clinicians, when asked to emulate the machine by classifying 10-sec EEG epochs out of context, would lose confidence in their judgment that a particular allocation was correct. Thus, suspicions are raised.

The EEG during sleep is remarkable for the range of variation it manifests for just one person and one night of sleep. Indeed, the EEG stages of alertness appear rather monotonous in comparison to the EEG stages of sleep. It is the great extremes of activity and the apparently fine gradations between them that motivate a desire for summarization (i.e., data reduction). This report is aimed at the application of data analysis for just such a purpose. We begin with a statement of the analysis problem and a discussion of the analysis objectives which emphasizes a comparison of discriminant and cluster analysis. This discussion is followed by a brief description of some problems common to cluster-seeking routines and a new clustering algorithm devised by one of the authors (EHR) which appears to be an attractive alternative to conventional clustering methods. This section is followed by a discussion of the physiological problem (EEG stages of sleep) and a presentation of experimental results from studies using the method previously described.

II. ANALYSIS PROBLEM

The analytic problem is twofold: to provide a means of description for the EEG itself, and then to systematize the resulting sets of measurements by recognizing patterns of measurements as members of some classification scheme. The patterns to be recognized may be categorized by prior knowledge of some classification scheme, or the scheme itself may be the result of a separate analysis.

The general problem of EEG analysis during sleep involves the problem of measurement as well as subsequent analysis of the selected measures. Insofar as the EEG is a time-varying voltage, the choice of measurement methods may include any one of a number of techniques for time series analysis. (The word "series" implies a discrete or digital representation of the signal although many possibilities exist for the analysis of continuous functions of time by analog methods.) The methods of measurement are critically important since all subsequent analysis is ultimately limited by the "information" contained in the set of measurements provided. Although each particular setting imposes unique constraints on the choice of measurement methods, we prefer frequency-based methods which provide a parcellation of the time series' total mean power into frequency bands with amplitude or intensity measures for each band such that the sum of the spectral intensities equal the total mean power of the time series.[1] The

---

[1] Total mean power is the mean squared value for the time function. This is a quadratic summary statistic which is analogous to a variance when the DC component is zero. The word power is taken from communications engineering where it is applied to an expenditure of energy. Total mean power is defined by

$$\bar{\psi}(x) = \frac{1}{T} \int_0^T x^2(t)dt.$$

The parcellation of power into frequencies is analogous to components of variance model. The summation properties are a classical result of Fourier series known as Parseval's theorum. Its statement is as follows:

$$\sum_{\infty}^{\infty} |c_n|^2/4 = \bar{\psi}(x) \text{ where } c_n \text{ is a complex Fourier coefficient } c = (a_n - ib_n)$$

where a_n and b_n are the cosine and sine coefficients of the series expansion. The quantity being summed can be related to the spectrum by noting the Fourier transformation (two-sided) of the sine wave $A \sin (\omega t + \phi)$ has two lines; one at $+\omega$, one at $-\omega$, each with amplitude $A/2$. Squaring to get the (two-sided) power spectrum gives $(A/2)^2$ or $A^2/4$. The indexes are for the two-sided spectrum.

reasons for this choice are based partly on conviction and partly on conclusion. A point of conclusion comes from an earlier study (Larsen and Walter, 1970), where it was shown that spectral representation of EEG selected by the APSS scoring criteria can provide sufficient "information" to allow successful recognition of sleep stages by numerical methods.

Another conclusion comes from the fact that a considerable body of sampling theory for both point and interval estimation is available for both auto and cross-spectral analysis. A comparable body of theory is not available for other methods of measurement.

A point of mathematical conclusion but physiological conviction comes from the fact that spectral analysis provides a more complete description of the time series than either interval measurements or their central tendencies. (Also, the latter are estimates of the moments of the spectrum.) Spectral analysis is related directly to the amplitude of the time series by Parseval's theorum, whereas period analysis is insensitive to absolute amplitudes. This is still only conviction physiological peaking because of correlations between interval measurements and amplitude in the EEG. The role of measurement is determined entirely by the objectives of the data analysis. In some situations, the best measurement is the adequate one. However, when measuring in uncertainty, the most important considerations may be precision, theoretical tractability, and completeness, which is merely a way of saying that brain/behavior correlation based on EEG is more likely to be fruitful as EEG measurement becomes more comprehensive. Thus conviction derives from simple notions that sufficient intensity in certain frequency bands does allow prediction (albeit imperfect) of the behavioral and visceral state of the intact animal.[2,3]

The relative advantages and deficiences of various measurement methods are discussed elsewhere in this volume, but it is well to keep in mind that

---

[2] A classical area of contention arising from this statement is the so-called behavioral EEG dissocation produced by systemic administration of atropine. In such situations, the EEG is slowed with increased amplitude to resemble a sleep-like state. The dissociation comes from the fact that by gross standards the animal is awake with a slowed EEG. However, humans given atropine as a preanesthetic medication report a twilight sleep condition rather unlike either arousal or unconscious sleep. Also, detailed psychological studies (*see* Longo, 1966, for a review) show atropine-related impairment in many behavioral situations. In fact, there is disruption of acquisition in operant and maze situations as well as a resistance to extinction. Atropine also may disrupt performance of a previously learned, rewarded behavior with the degree of disruption proportional to the EEG synchronization (Sadowski and Longo, 1962).

[3] A particularly interesting method by which to study psychophysiological correlates of EEG states defined by frequency content is to produce long trains of a particular rhythm by operant conditioning with simultaneous recording of relevant physiological parameters. Examples of this include EEG, cardiovascular, and respiratory changes in two variates of transcendental meditation, Zen and Yoga, and recent studies with conditioning the sensorimotor rhythm (*cf.* Tart, 1969, and Harper and Chase, *in preparation*).

this choice is the information-limiting step. Constructive insight at this stage of the data analysis may provide the great benefit of allowing simplication of subsequent treatment. How much the problem can be simplified and still retain its meaning is another question.

Discriminant Analysis[4] and Cluster Analysis

The logical distinctions between discriminant analysis and cluster analysis are important in the design of a data analysis system for automation of clinical electroencepholography. By virtue of this fact, some preliminary discussion of the notions involved and attention to the terminology may be useful. A measurement is a numerical description of some feature which we deem an important aspect of the EEG. In the case of spectral analysis, the measurement is an intensity at some center frequency for a given spectral window shape and width. This may be standardized to a 1-Hz resolution which defines the spectral density function. Its ordinates are the portion of total average power contributed by components in the frequency range ω to $\omega + \Delta\omega$ about some center value.

In a typical EEG spectrum calculated at 1-Hz resolution over the band 1 to 32 Hz, the set of 32 spectral intensities constitute an ordered array of measurements. The set of these measurements corresponds to a point on a 32 dimensional space by virtue of a Cartesian co-ordinate system in the same way a set of three numbers locates a point in three-dimensional space through a three-dimensional rectangular co-ordinate system; that is, one axis is assigned to each spectral ordinate. Thus, the spectral intensity in each band becomes itself a variate whose behavior is studied by observing that spectral intensity for a sample of EEG epochs. Taken alone, each variate has a distribution of cases over its range of values. In this way a histogram can be made which describes the behavior of the variate results. When two ordinates in the spectrum are considered simultaneously, each EEG epoch has associated with it values for two variates. A Cartesian co-ordinate system with two dimensions then establishes a correspondence between the pair of numbers and a geometrical point in a two-dimensional space. As all EEG samples are "plotted" in the space, a scatter diagram is formed. The two variates have some pairs of values which occur in the sample more often than other pairs of values. A systematic representation of this aspect of their simultaneous behavior becomes a generalization of the histogram

---

[4]The meaning we apply to discriminant analysis is that of a genera of analytic techniques for classifying observations into two or more *a priori* groups. We are not limiting the term to the parametrically determined discriminant function of Fisher or the multigroup (also parametric) extension due to Rao.

concept to a bivariate joint distribution. Similarly, in the 32-dimensional situation, it takes 32 axes to establish a correspondence between an array of 32 variate values and a geometrical point in a 32 dimensional space. The variates taken alone still have univariate (marginal) distributions, and they also have a joint distribution for all 32 variates as well as a variety of conditional distributions. Both cluster analysis and discriminant analysis operate in this multivariate space; but this part of the discussion is reserved for later sections.

The set of numbers, or alternatively the geometrical point, constitute a pattern of measurements.[5] When the process of measurement is repeatedly applied to EEG samples, a swarm of geometrical points will result. Algebraically, the result is a set of arrays (patterns), each one of which is itself a set of measurements. The problem now progresses to classifying the set of patterns. In the language of artificial intelligence, this is a pattern classification and its aim is data reduction. That is, instead of having, for example, 100 points representing 100 "groups" of EEGs, we would like some definition of grouping which would aggregate, say, 10 of the samples into type A, 30 of the samples into type B, and so forth. We have accomplished data reduction because we now can describe the 100 EEG segments in terms of, hopefully, a small number of groups instead of 100 groups of size one. Presumably, patterns should be similar within a group and dissimilar between groups. At this point, two of the difficulties with cluster analysis become apparent: (1) how does one decide on the number of groups, and (2) how is the classification system to be defined and what constraints should be placed on the groups which result? Since no generally satisfying solution exists to these problems, one is usually forced into an *ad hoc,* empirical approach. Even given this, the entire result may be altered by normalization and scaling of measurements. Lastly, one is usually interested in how the groups relate as the number of groups increase and diminish. Perhaps, at this point an illustration from taxonomy may be helpful. Given a sample of insects from each of a large number of regions on Earth, how does one define species, and, once this is determined, how do the species relate to genera, the genera to families, and so forth (*cf.* Sokal and Sneath, 1963).

When the problem is one of numerical classification, one can think of abstract machines which "look" at patterns and sort them into categories. This pattern classifying machine may be "trained" to recognize patterns as members of certain groups and sort them in some way which minimizes errors of allocation. Thus, in a sense the machine has learned to recognize

---

[5] As a pedagogic device, it may be said that a particular sample of EEG represents a pattern of EEG activity such as alert-eyes-closed α, sleep spindles or the like. Thus, a sample of an EEG pattern becomes a pattern of numbers by way of the process of measurement.

patterns as members of groups. Defining the groups or discovering a classification system is the business of cluster analysis. Once the groups are defined, sorting patterns into the "correct" group is the business of discriminant analysis. A learning machine which finds the groups and sorts the individual patterns into the groups so determined is said to be unsupervised; a learning machine which sorts cases into a given system of classification is said to be supervised. The former employs cluster analysis and discriminant analysis, the latter only discriminant analysis (*cf.* Nilsson, 1965).

The term cluster analysis is meant to describe a genera of analytic methods (see Ball, 1965, for review) for the discovery of a classification system. The objective is to map similar observations into the same set with dissimilar observations in different sets. Within this broad requirement many operational varieties are possible according to the constraints and measures of similarity which may be used. Typical measures of similarity include correlations and distances. These constitute the fundamental datum on which the cluster analysis operates. The next requirement is to define a measure of cluster quality. This is accomplished by providing constraints for the properties of the resulting groups. Then the process must "find" a solution which in some sense is optimal in terms of the constraints. Hill-climbing methods of optimization require reevaluation of the cluster result each time a point is moved to a new set or the number of sets changes as the quality of the final outcome must depend on the disposition of each point in respect to the disposition of every other point. Iterative cluster analysis techniques are consequently infamous as great consumers of CPU time.

Before considering the particular method of Ruspini (1969), it is prudent to display some of the relevant problems affecting cluster analysis routines. For example, distance measures are very sensitive to normalization and scaling. Rather different clustering can result from the same data by altering these adjuncts to measurement. As an illustration, consider the following figure taken from Ball (1965). Ball points out that *moderate* (the italics are Ball's) normalization, scaling, and linear transformation are likely to have little effect if well-defined clusters exist in the data. However, when the clusters are disputable, the results may depend intimately on the particular scaling and transformation procedures employed.

Also, in methods using distance as the primary datum, the choice of distance metric will clearly exert a profound effect on the cluster result. This effect is illustrated in Fig. 2, taken from Ball (1965), where the grouping is entirely different depending on whether the distance is a likelihood or a distance from the centroid.

Also, Nagy (1968) has detailed several difficulties that lead to classifications which place similar points in different sets; these compromising situ-

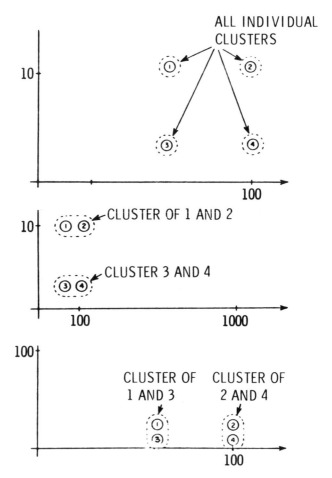

FIG. 1. Effect of measurement scaling on clustering (from Ball, 1965).

ations are illustrated in Fig. 3, taken from his publication. Lastly, there is the problem of determining the number of groups. Changing the number of groups frequently produces compromising situations of the type detailed by Nagy. Illustrations of this effect and unequal cluster density are taken from Ruspini (Fig. 4 and 5).

The particular method developed by Ruspini (1969, 1970) avoids some of the difficulties due to stray and bridge cases by clustering a fuzzy set. Fuzzy sets (Zadah, 1962) are sets for which a degree of belongingness is allowed. Rather than a point being in or out of a set (the conventional situation), a

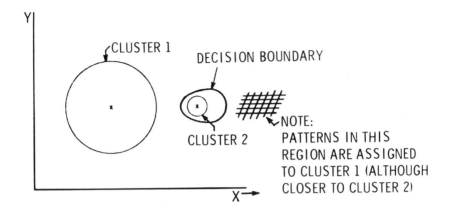

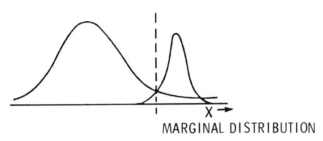

FIG. 2. Effect of distance metric on cluster assignment by minimum distance. Cases in the cross-hatched region would be assigned to cluster 1 if the metric were based on likelihoods, but they would be assigned to cluster 2 if the metric were based on distance (Euclidian) from the centroid (from Ball, 1965).

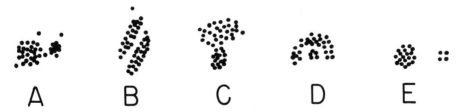

FIG. 3. The major difficulties found in cluster analysis are illustrated by the following: A and C demonstrate bridge cases between clusters; B illustrates nonspherical clusters; D shows clusters which are not linearly separable; and E illustrates unequal prior probabilities (from Nagy, 1968).

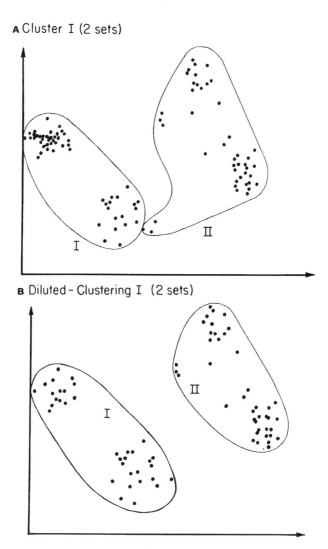

A Cluster I (2 sets)

B Diluted - Clustering I (2 sets)

FIG. 4. Effect of unequal cluster density. In a, the dense region in the upper part of I causes three points to be anomalously contained in II. A dilution of all cases, as shown in b, allows the two sets to have convex hulls (from Ruspini, 1969).

point may belong to a set to a greater or lesser degree. Stray and bridge cases are in the fuzzy regions with a degree of belonging near zero, whereas cases near the core may belong to the set with a degree of one. Ruspini places this notion in a probabilistic setting by virtue of the fact that the clustering process decomposes the data set density function into a linear

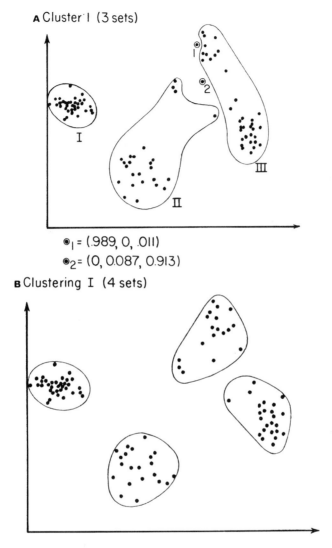

FIG. 5. Effect of the number of available sets. In particular, note the two fuzzy points in the three-set situation and the satisfying product with four sets (from Ruspini, 1969).

combination of component cluster (set) densities, $P(x|S_j)$, and prior probabilities, $P(S_j)$. That is, $P(x) = \Sigma_j P(S_j)P(x|S_j)$. The component set densities are interpreted as representing the degree of belongingness of each point to each cluster, and the prior probabilities are measures of the size of each set. The decomposition is performed subject to the constraint that the average mean square distance of a point to the class it most likely belongs is mini-mized. This is intended to insure that the component density functions really do represent clusters. That is, the following quadratic quanity is minimized (the notion is after Ruspini, 1969):

$$\sum_{i=1}^{i}[P(x_i)P(S_{(i)})M_{(i)}(x_i)/M(x_i)]$$

where the sum is over all cases, $P(x_i)$ is the density function evaluated for case i, $P(S_{(i)})$ is the prior probability for the most like set, $M_{(i)}(x_i)$ is the mean density of the most likely set around case i, and $M(x_i)$ is the mean density of the population around x_i. The circled points in Fig. 5b are cases in fuzzy regions of the sets. The numbers indicate degrees of belongingness, in terms of conditional probabilities $P(S_j|x_j)$, for each of the possible sets.

III. THE PHYSIOLOGICAL PROBLEM

The primal question is, "What does the EEG do during sleep?" The quick-est answer is that it does a great deal. In fact, it does so much that some method of summarization (i.e., data reduction) is necessary to avoid being swamped by the volume and variety of EEG produced by the sleeping brain. The efforts of clinical electroencephalographers over decades have resulted in at least two systems of classification based on the powerful pattern-classi-fying capacity for two-dimensional images indigenous to the human CNS. When this is combined with an equally powerful capacity for pattern recog-nition of two-dimensional images, one may wonder what the computer has to offer. One easily appreciated computer application is to relieve the sleep researcher from the tedium of scoring vast quantities of EEG records. Machine service as a human substitute for such tasks raises many inter-esting and important questions of its own in addition to freeing the scientist or clinician or both for more original work. Whereas this is important and necessary, the present chapter is addressed more to the use of automation to extend our concepts about what the EEG does during sleep. The task is prodigious, even by computer standards, since a single night of sleep may produce an 8-hr tape containing 16 channels of information. If one were to digitize (for the DC to 100 Hz bandwidth) and analyze all of it, this would represent something like 100 million data points to be processed for only one night and one subject. It is, in part, from the sheer enormity of the task that clinical pattern classification and pattern recognition must operate on a fairly long time base with substantial degrees of averaging, smoothing, and inertia in the output of the human "learning machine." Whereas this has added enormously significant findings to our knowledge of sleep and its related processes, one must wonder if the loss of information may be a source of conceptual prejudice. This may become especially cogent when one observes that a 3-minute epoch named stage 3 by the rules of the Association for the Psychophysiological Study of Sleep may contain periods which are clearly not even slow-wave sleep. Incursions of REM-like periods in predominantly slow wave epochs and the brief appearance of slow wave periods in predominantly REM or light sleep epochs may have great relevance for quantitative studies of sleep stage deprivation and rebound. These incursion phenomena raise further questions of electro-clinical correlation. Given that a subject is well into stage 4 sleep (with some defined strength of stimulus necessary for arousal), what importance may be attributed to a 10 sec period clearly not stage 4? Have thresholds to arousal changed during that 10 seconds? Is this a micro example of EEG/behavioral dissociation? More germane to the present paper, however, is the question of how a cluster analysis of the EEG during sleep might suggest modifications to our concepts of EEG stages of sleep. Most students of sleep would admit that the APSS sleep staging system is, to some extent, an artifice. Nevertheless, few researchers would confidently delimit the degree of appropriate or inappropriate misrepresentation so imposed. A major purpose of this study is to help provide the design and devices which may prove useful in examining this sort of physiological question.

Before embarking on a sketch of the experimental design and a presentation of results, it is relevant to consider the particular experimental setting (see Larsen, Walter, McNew, and Adey, *in press,* for details). The experimental animals were two unrestrained chimpanzees from whom analog signals were telemetered to a receiver and subsequently recorded on analog FM magnetic tape. The two animals were used as replications of within-subject analyses rather than pooling data from two sources. The sole source of data for numerical analysis is one channel of EEG derived from a bipolar arrangement consisting of parietal and right occipital skull screws. After digitizing, the time series was subjected to spectral analysis as performed by computer program BMD X92 (Dixon, 1969). Thus, 32 spectral ordinates (at 1 Hz resolution, centered on integer frequencies, over the band, 1 to 32 Hz) served as a description of each EEG sample. The single analysis channel was supplemented by hippocampal EEG, EOG, and EMG for purposes of clinical classification.

A. Discrimination Testing

The experimental design begins with a test of a sleep classification system with the following categories: Drowsy, Light, Medium, Deep, and REM (see McNew, Kado, Howe, Zweizig, and Adey, 1968, for details). The test proceeded by means of a training/testing paradigm with parametric discriminant analysis as performed by computer program BMD 07M (Dixon, 1968). That is, approximately 100 EEG samples were selected from distributed segments of the record which sampled periods thought to be unequivocal examples of each sleep stage. Thus, each sleep stage was represented by approximately 20 samples taken by a stratified design. This process was repeated for each of the two animals, but with two standards within the strata. In the first animal, Dinky, only samples very close to an idealized picture of the EEG for each stage were accepted. In the second animal, Kelly, the qualifications were relaxed to allow expression of the range of variation in each EEG stage. Discriminant functions were generated within each animal on the basis of this preclustered data. Thus discriminant functions were applied to the classification of EEG epochs that were new data. The former set is known as training data according to the learning machine paradigm previously described. The new data do not enter into the generation of the discriminant functions and are the testing data set. Error rates are estimated on the test data in order to reduce bias (see Larsen, Walter, McNew, and Adey, *in press*). Most importantly, the test data did not reflect any particular classification system; in fact, the test data were gathered by a systematic sampling design which took the first 10 sec of every 6 min of EEG record throughout the night of sleep.[6] This process will represent EEG epochs in proportion to their probability of occurrence. This is important for two reasons. (1) It contrasts with the stratified sampling in the training data where the probability of sampling a particular region of EEG depends on some epoch's similarity to an archetype, and the probability of sampling a stratum does not depend on the prior probability of the stratum. (2) The error rates in the test set will reflect misclassifications from clusters with high prior probabilities more than it will epochs from clusters with low prior probabilities.

Each of these systematic samples was classified according to the LMD system by clinical judgment. Approximately 120 periods were available from each animal to form this category of test data. (As a mnemonic aid, these data will be identified as non-preclustered, or NPC, test data.)

The objective is to estimate error rates for test data classified by means of discriminant functions generated on training data selected according to two realizations of the LMD sleep classification system. It is extended to examine the proposition that handling transition epochs is the major short-

---

[6] A random sample may have been preferable, but it was felt that the systematic sampling was unlikely to synchronize with some unknown sleep cycling process with a 6-min period. Even if such cycles exist, it seems unlikely that they would be clocked independently of arousals and awakenings.

coming of conventional sleep-staging systems. This is accomplished by means of the two standards for entrance into the training data set. In the first case, conservative sampling resulted in minimal within-group variation and close similarity to an idealized picture of the EEG in each stage. In the second case, liberalized requirements allowed the training set to reflect the range of variation within each stage. To the extent that the latter system corresponds more closely with clusters in the NPC test data (i.e., it is a more "realistic" training set), the error rates in the NPC test data would be lower than the idealized training set[7] (unless the liberalized training set itself is grossly unclustered, which is not the case as evidenced by the discriminant space plots in Fig. 7). The end stage would, of course, be a training set which was not preclustered at all. This is exactly the situation studied by cluster analysis in unsupervised learning.

In addition, this design allows for an epoch-by-epoch examination of errors in the testing data set. This information is useful in delimiting the nature of the misrepresentation imposed by the training set classification system.

These discriminations were informative in two regards. (1) When conservative archetypes served as the training data and these data were plotted in a two-dimensional reduced discriminant space[8] along with the test data,

---

[7] Note that this method can proceed only by exclusion. We can "test" for the absence of a classification system, but the finding of low error rates cannot serve as evidence that a training set classification system is a correct (i.e., in some sense optimal) representation of clusters in the data.

This approach is limited further by the methods of discrimination employed. To the extent that nonlinear or nonparametric methods would give lower error rates, we would commit a type II error by declaring the training set classification system as untenable. These notes are intended to emphasize a lack of power and the need for true cluster analysis to complete the picture available from discrimination.

[8] A discriminant space representation is a linear transformation of the training data into a new coordinate system. This coordinate system is, in general, the same dimensionality as the test space. That is, a p dimensional discriminant space is constructed by forming p linear combinations of the test space variates. Each linear combination defines a composite variable, and each variate is associated with a discriminant space coordinate axis. The first discriminant space (canonical) variate is derived to maximize the ratio of between to within groups variance for cases in the training set. The second canonical variate is constrained to be uncorrelated with the first, but to be the one linear combination which maximizes the same ratio. Subsequent variates are likewise mutually uncorrelated, each determined by the linear combination which provides the variate with the largest possible value of the criterion. As criterion values decrease, one may select a subset which contains the r largest values. When the sum of the first k criterion values are large compared to the sum of all p criterion values, the result is dimensionality reduction with often only slight loss discrimination power. Mathematically, the weights we seek for the linear combinations are found to be the vectors invariant under the linear transformation $[W^{-1}A]$ where W^{-1} is the inverse of the within-groups matrix of cross products of deviations and A is the among or between groups matrix of cross products of deviations. The criterion values are the eigen values of the determental equation $|W^{-1}A - \lambda X| = 0$. The first axis is determined by the eigen vector associated with the largest eigen value, the second axis by the next-to-largest value, and so on.

it was apparent that the training set occupies a very small region compared to the test cases. In fact, approximately 50% of the test cases are entirely off-scale for both SYNC and DESYNC subsets (see Fig. 6). Error rates in the NPC test data are rather high at about 30% overall.[9]

When liberalized archetypes serve as training data, the RDS plots show that the training set covers much more of the range of variation, as shown in Fig. 7. However, NPC test set error rates are essentially unchanged at approximately 30% misclassifications overall.

In addition, the vast majority of test errors with the conservative training set were due to test cases remote from any archetype case. In other words, the majority of misclassified test cases were dissimilar from any training set case. The liberalized archetypes represented the test data range of variation to a dramatically improved extent. However, the continued high error rate belies a still substantial degree of misrepresentation which was not reduced by including the group tails (see Table 1). In fact, Kelly's SNYC subset plot discloses substantial numbers of transition cases, which suggests that the liberalized SYNC training set still represents clusters with far more distinctness than are present in the test data.

In summary, these discriminations lead us to the following conclusions.

(1) Conservative archetypes do not cover the range of variation in the NPC test data to any realistic extent.[10]

(2) Error rates in the NPC test data are quite similar for both degrees of archetype (training data) preclustering. The implication is that neither training set expression of the LMD classification system constitutes discriminable clusters in the NPC testing data.

(3) Although Kelly's training set covered most of the range of variation seen in the testing data set (compare Figs. 1 and 2), the test data error rates were rather high at approximately 30% overall. One would have expected that liberalized requirements for archetype admission would reduce error rates to the extent that transition epochs were being misclassified. The results again lead to the implication that if clusters do exist in the NPC test data, they do not coincide with those in even a liberalized version of the LMD classification system (as far as one can judge by the discrimination methods herein applied).

---

[9] Error rates are tabulated according to the subset and decision layer in which they occur. They are not tabulated according to groups because this is inconsistent with the systematic sampling.

[10] As might be expected, a training/testing design with test data as an archetype subset produced much lower error rates at the DESYNC/SYNC discrimination with conservative archetypes than with liberal archtypes. Error rates in the latter situation were about twice those in the former (Larsen et al., *in preparation*).

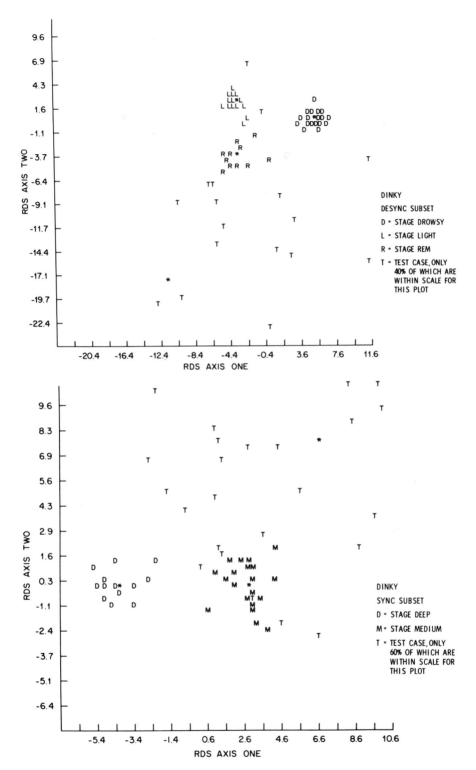

FIG. 6. Plots of training and test cases in a two-dimensional reduced discriminant space for Dinky's DESYNC and SYNC subsets.

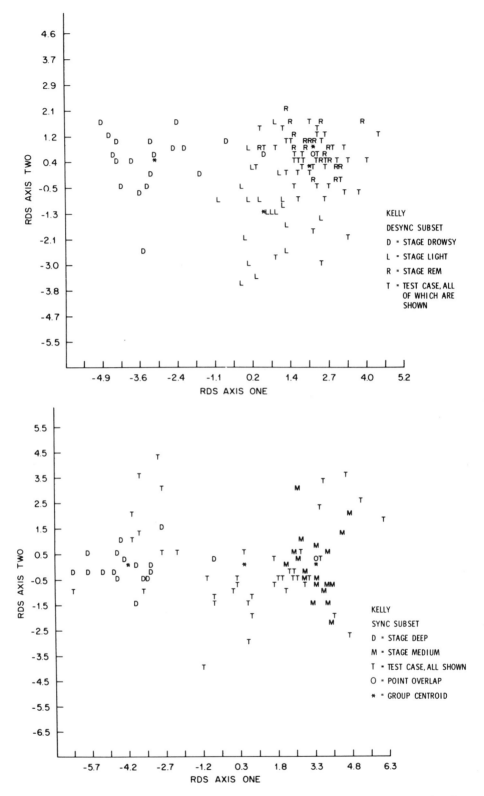

FIG. 7. Plots of training and test cases in reduced discriminant space for Kelly's DESYNC and SYNC subsets.

TABLE 1. Error rates for discrimination of NPC test data by archetype training data

	Dinky		Kelly	
	DESYNC	SYNC	DESYNC	SYNC
Layer 1 **SYNC-DESYNC discrimination**				
Train	0%	0%	0%	0%
Test over-all subsets	22% (7/32)	16% (14/81) 19% (21/113)	8% (3/38)	15.6% (10/64) 12.8% (13/102)
Layer II **DESYNC and SYNC** [subsets separately considered with new errors (Test) and all errors (Layers I and II)]				
Test	20% (5/32–7)	10.5% (7/81–14)	34% (12/38–2)	5.6% (3/64–10)
Layers I and II (overall subsets and layers)	38% (12/32)	26% (12/81) 29% (33/113)	40% (15/38)	20% (13/64) 27% (28/102)

(4) The better coverage provided by the liberalized archetypes still left substantial numbers of outlyers and bridge cases in the NPC test data.

(5) When counting every disagreement between machine and clinical allocation as an error, many misclassified test cases were remote from any of the archetype cases for the "correct" group. This was true for both degrees of archetype preclustering, although it was more frequently the case with Dinky's data.

(6) The RDS plots of Kelly's SYNC subset affirm the artificiality of the Medium/Deep (or Stage 3/Stage 4) distinction.

(7) The RDS plots of Kelly's DESYNC subset confirm the distinctness of stage Drowsy from the loose combination of stages Light and REM (due to the rhythmic alpha ?).

Cluster Analysis of EEG During Sleep

Verification of the Algorithm. Even though Cluster I has been the object of extensive numerical experiments (Ruspini, 1970), we felt it would be prudent to test the algorithm on the type of data to which it would be applied. The data most suitable for this purpose are Dinky's archetype set where both the number and the nature of the clusters was set by conservative clinical selection. Cluster analysis of this data based on the previously described spectral representation sorted the preclustered data as shown in Table 2. This result was felt to be rather unsatisfactory (especially in its handling of REM, Light, and Medium), which led to a reconsideration of the problems of normalization and scaling. The procedure adopted was based on a principal components analysis of the correlation matrix for the 32 variates on 100 observations. The first five axes of the new coordinate system were preserved for later analysis.[11] This, of course, effected a dimensionality reduction as well as a rescaling of the data. Euclidian distances in this new five-dimensional space then served as input for the clustering algorithm. The results are shown in Table 2. It is apparent that Cluster I operated much better on the rescaled and linearly transformed variates than it did on the raw variate; this is evidenced particularly in REM, Light, Medium, and Deep by the percent of cases falling into the largest cluster: REM, 100%; Light, 70%; Medium, 64%; and Deep, 100%; compared to 64%, 50%, 50%, and 70%, respectively, for the raw data.

---

[11]That is, the data were mapped into a new space by linear transformation $[A^*]$ where $[A^*]$ is the first five columns of the unrotated factor pattern matrix.

$$[X]_{100.32}[A^*]_{32.5} = [X^*]_{100.5}$$

The first five eigen values of $[R]$ accounted for 80 to 85% of the trace. As a mnemonic aid, the transformed variates will also be referred to as orthogonalized.

TABLE 2. Comparison of cluster location for Dinky's archetype data in five sets with raw and orthogonalized variates

	Orthogonal	Raw
REM	C_2, 11/11	C_2, 7/11; C_5, 3/11; C_3, 1/11
Drowsy	C_5, 16/22; C_4, 6/22	C_4, 20/22; $C_{5.2}$, 1/22 each
Light	C_3, 14/20; C_2, 4/20; $C_{1.5}$, 1/20 each	C_2, 10/20; C_4, 10/20
Medium	C_4, 14/22; C_2, 4/22; $C_{1.5}$, 2/22 each	C_5, 11/22; C_3, 9/22; $C_{1.2}$, 1/22 each
Deep	C_1, 14/14	C_1, 11/14; C_3, 3/14

In conclusion, the transformed data cluster in ways more consistent with prior knowledge of archetype composition. We also conclude that Cluster I is capable of detecting clusters in this sort of sleep data after transformation as above. In further discussion, all distances will be computed after transformation unless otherwise specified.

C. Cluster Analysis of the NPC Test Data

After the operation of Cluster I on preclustered data was verified, the algorithm was applied to Dinky's NPC test data. For purposes of comparing the clinical classification of each test epoch with the cluster analysis result, the number of clusters was set at five. The results of this analysis and our present interpretation of them are in Fig. 8.

The results suggest two primary clusters labeled synchronous (SYNC) and desynchronous (DESYNC), corresponding to the gross appearance of the EEG. This is similar in concept to the SYNC and DESYNC clusters

	Cluster I	Cluster II	Cluster III	Cluster IV (SYNC)	Cluster V
Deep, Dm	0	0	1	5	8
D/M, M/D	0	0	2	4	6
Medium	9	6	10 [MEDIUM]	14	1
M/L, L/M, M/R	6	3	2	1	0
Light, L/Dr	0	2	1	1	0
Drowsy, Dr/R	0	1	1	0	0
REM, R/M, R/Dr	9 [DESYNC]	3	9	0	3

FIG. 8. Cluster analysis of Dinky's NPC data in five sets.

identified by Larsen and Walter (1970) in a previous human study. In that study Stages 2, 3, and 4 occupied the SYNC subset, whereas Stages Wake, 1, and REM occupied the DESYNC subset. In the present study, Stage Medium includes Stage 2 plus the "lighter half" of Stage 3; deeper levels of Stage 3 and all of Stage 4 constitute stage Deep. As shown in Fig. 8, Medium cases are prominent contributors to both SYNC and DESYNC clusters. The implication is that Stage Medium bridges the two clusters. This is similar to the finding that DESYNC and SYNC clusters were bridged by cases from Stages 1 and 2 in the earlier study (Larsen and Walter, 1970).

Further evidence that these clusters do exist is gained from the fact that percentualization of the spectral ordinates (a normalizing operation) before the components analysis gave essentially unchanged results. (There may be a slight benefit to the nonpercentual spectra because Deep and D/M cases are more compactly distributed over the available sets) (see Fig. 9).

	Cluster II	Cluster III	Cluster V	Cluster IV	Cluster I
Deep, Dm	I	I	I	5	6
D/M, M/D	I	3	O	8	I
Medium	2	7	7	16	8
M/L, M/R	2	4	2	O	I
Light, L/Dr, L/M	2	2	2	O	I
Drowsy, Dr/R	I	O	O	O	I
REM, R/M, R/Dr	I3	3	6	I	I

FIG. 9. Cluster results with the preceding data and percentual spectra.

When the analysis was repeated for Kelly's NPC test data, the same picture emerges (Fig. 10).

Normalizing the spectra before transformation gave essentially unchanged results except for slightly fewer stray cases. In both animals, the most compact regions in the clusters are associated with groups Deep and REM (Fig. 11).

It seems reasonable to conclude, therefore, that the most reliable estimate of the structure underlying the NPC test data is that of two diffuse aggregates—SYNC and DESYNC with Medium cases occupying both subsets.

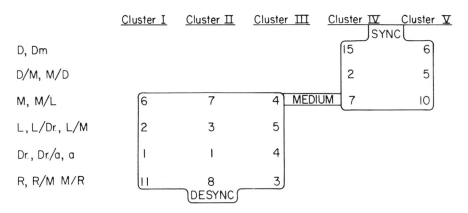

	Cluster I	Cluster II	Cluster IV (SYNC)	Cluster III	Cluster V
Deep, Dm	2	O	1	6	12
D/M, M/D	1	1	3	0	2
Medium, M/L, M/R	6	5	MEDIUM 13	7	5
L, L/Dr, L/M	4	5	0	1	0
Dr., Dr./a, a	4	2	1	0	1
R, R/M	6	9 (DESYNC)	2	3	0

FIG. 10. Kelly's NPC test data in five sets.

	Cluster I	Cluster II	Cluster III	Cluster IV (SYNC)	Cluster V
D, Dm				15	6
D/M, M/D				2	5
M, M/L	6	7	4 MEDIUM	7	10
L, L/Dr, L/M	2	3	5		
Dr., Dr./a, a	1	1	4		
R, R/M M/R	11	8 (DESYNC)	3		

FIG. 11. Cluster results with the preceding data and percentual spectra.

Within these two diffuse clusters, the most compact regions were associated with groups Deep and REM.[12]

IV. COMMENT

One physiological interpretation of these two diffuse clusters, each one with a slightly dense region, is that the majority of cases in the NPC test

---

[12] This impression is strengthened by a cluster analysis of Kelly's combined archetype and NPC test data. The only test groups showing even a modest degree of concordance in cluster location were REM and Deep. This concordance persisted with percentual spectra (Larsen et al., *in preparation*).

data are a mixture of two generating systems. The dense regions may be the relatively pure product of one generating system, whereas the generally diffuse nature of the clusters is the result of combining the two systems in various proportions. Further, the rapid switching of EEG state, as demonstrated by an analysis of discrimination errors, implies a fluttering, dynamic relationship between the two generating systems.

Qualifications to this analysis include the following: (1) the data source is limited to a spectral analysis of one EEG channel; (2) EEG recorded from the surface of the cortex is less stable and generally more active in the beta region of the spectrum than scalp-recorded EEG which receives greater spatial averaging and signal filtering; (3) the results although consistent are from only two animals; (4) larger sample sizes in both archetype and systematically sampled data sets may be needed (although this study employed nearly 400 EEG epochs).

This enumeration of qualifications is not intended to suggest an incredulity to the results; rather it is intended to emphasize that cluster analysis of sleep is in the infancy of its development. All manner of experimental and analytic conditions affect the results in ways that are not easily predictable. This class of analysis is hazardous and challenging to a degree exceeding most other types of multivariate analysis. By design, cluster analysis lacks the prior information usually available to data analysis. This is at once its major source of interest and its major source of consternation.

V. SUMMARY

General conclusions from the discrimination and cluster analysis are that the LMD sleep staging system does not closely represent clusters in systematically sampled (not preclustered or NPC) test data. Furthermore, liberalizing the range of variation in the training set left error rates in the NPC test data unchanged. This, combined with the cluster analysis of the NPC test data, leaves the impression that the most reliable estimate of the underlying structure in the NPC data set is two diffuse clusters. These are labeled DESYNC and SYNC on the basis of the gross appearance of the contributing EEGs. The two clusters are most compact in regions corresponding to groups Deep and REM, and Medium cases occupy both subsets.

DISCUSSION

Larsen was congratulated for his general exposition of the way in which cluster analysis techniques could be applied to a particular problem in EEG.

Criticisms raised by the discussants pertained mainly to the limitations of the extent to which conclusions could be drawn from this particular experiment. For example, Larsen agreed that this study showed only that this particular way of examining sleep EEG, namely a technique employing spectral analysis, did not result in identification of categories corresponding to the Dement-Kleitman stages of sleep which have been formally defined by the Association for the Psychophysiological Study of Sleep. Further qualification to this analysis raised by some of the discussants are considered by the authors in the *Comment* section of their paper.

ACKNOWLEDGMENTS

Computations performed by the Data Processing Laboratory of the Brain Research Institute were supported in part by U.S. Public Health Service grant NB–02501. Computations performed at the Health Sciences Computing Facility were supported by National Institutes of Health grant FR–3.

The author is a recipient of a postdoctoral National Institutes of Health (extramural) fellowship #1 F2 NB 39, 931–01 NSRB.

It is a pleasure to acknowledge patient assistance in typing and figure preparation by Mrs. L. Mayer and the Medical Illustration Department, respectively, of the Walter Reed Army Institute of Research.

REFERENCES

Ball, G. H. (1965): Data analysis in the social sciences: What about the details? *Proceedings of the Fall Joint Computer Conference*, pp. 533–559.
Dixon, W. J. (1965): *BMD Biomedical Computer Programs*. Health Sciences Computing Facility, UCLA School of Medicine, Los Angeles, Calif., 599 pp.
Dixon, W. J. (1969): *BMD Biomedical Computer Programs X-Series Supplement*. Health Sciences Computing Facility, UCLA School of Medicine, Los Angeles, Calif., 260 pp.
Larsen, L. E., and Walter, D. O. (1970): On automatic methods of sleep staging by EEG spectra. *Electroencephalography and Clinical Neurophysiology*, 28:459–467.
Larsen, L. E., Walter, D. O., McNew, J. J., and Adey, W. R. On the problem of bias in error rate estimation for discriminant analysis. *Pattern Recog. (in press)*.
Longo, V. G. (1966): Behavioral and electrographic effects of atropine and related compounds: *Pharmacological Reviews*, 18:965–996.
McNew, J. J., Kado, R. T., Howe, R. C., Zweizig, T. R., and Adey, W. R. (1968): Telemetry studies of sleep in the unrestrained chimpanzee. *Institute of Electrical and Electronics Engineers National Telemetering Conference Record*, pp. 374–381.
Nagy, G. (1968): State of the art in pattern recognition. *Proceedings of the Institute of Electrical and Electronics Engineers*, 56:836–882.
Nilsson, N. J. (1965): *Learning Machines: Foundations of Trainable Pattern-Classifying Machines*. McGraw-Hill, New York, 137 pp.
Ruspini, E. H. (1969): A new approach to clustering. *Information Control*, 15:22–32.
Ruspini, E. H. (1970): Numerical methods for fuzzy clustering. *Information Sciences*, 2:319–350.

Sadowski, B., and Longo, V. G. (1962): EEG and behavioral correlates of an instrumental reward conditioned response in rabbits. A physiological and pharmacological study. *Electroencephalography and Clinical Neurophysiology*, 14:465–476.

Sokal, R. R., and Sneath, P. H. A. (1963): *Principles of Numerical Taxonomy*. W. H. Freeman & Co., San Franciso.

Tart, C. T. (Ed.) (1969): *Altered States of Consciousness*. John Wiley, New York, Chapters 33 and 34.

Zadeh, L. A. (1965): Fuzzy sets. *Information Control*, 8:338–353.

Automation of Clinical Electroencephalography.
Edited by P. Kellaway and I. Petersén.
Raven Press, New York © 1973.

Automatic Analysis of the EEG for Sleep Staging

S. S. Viglione and W. B. Martin

Pattern Recognition Technology, Research and Development Directorate, McDonnell Douglas Astronautics Company, Huntington Beach, California

I. INTRODUCTION

The EEG recording has long served as a clinical aid for the diagnosis of epilepsy, mental disorders, and brain defects. More recently, the EEG has provided a tool for categorizing sleep periods of normal subjects. The EEG signal successively assumes several well-defined patterns throughout the course of a normal night's sleep. Dement and Kleitman (1957) classified these patterns into the following sleep states:

Stage 1 — Low-voltage signal with irregular frequency.
Stage 2 — 13 to 15 Hz sleep spindles and "K" complexes in a low voltage background.
Stage 3 — Sets of large delta waves (1 to 3 Hz) appear frequently.
Stage 4 — EEG composed almost entirely of delta waves.

Most subjects move through this succession of stages in the first hour of sleep. After Stage 4 sleep, the EEG returns to a low-voltage irregular waveform; this is accompanied by bursts of rapid eye movement (REM). This sleep stage has been termed Stage REM. During the rest of the sleep period the EEG tends to alternate between REM and Stage 2 in cycles ranging from 90 to 120 min. Figure 1 illustrates the sleep-stage transitions one could go through during a night's sleep. This record of sleep performance is referred to as a "sleep print." The categorization of sleep has led to more ac-

269

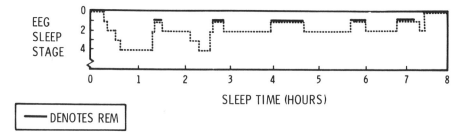

FIG. 1. Sleep print.

curate determination of various phenomena occurring during sleep; for example, a high correlation has been established between dreaming and the occurrence of Stage REM.

Researchers studying the relationships between sleep and psychological or physiological phenomena therefore rely heavily upon the EEG and the electro-oculograph (EOG) recordings in categorizing various sleep periods of normal human subjects. The present method of visually classifying EEG records in the awake and various sleep categories requires a great deal of time on the part of a skilled encephalographer. In addition, human scorers are not always consistent in interpreting the scoring rules for each sleep category. One objective of this research effort was, therefore, to develop and to improve systems or devices for identifying sleep stages automatically and, using the methods of pattern recognition technology, to put sleep scoring on a more quantitative basis.

To attack the problem, two broad approaches were attempted. The first involves performing a frequency analysis of the EEG, divided into short time epochs, and allowing a self-organizing pattern recognition system to associate the frequency information (spectrum) with sleep stages on a set of sample patterns previously classified by human scorers. If a representative sample of each sleep stage may be obtained and sufficient information is retained in the spectrum of the EEG, no knowledge of sleep patterns is required. The recognition system adaptively derives the appropriate correlations between the frequency information and the sleep state.

The second area of investigation, called Known Property Extraction, requires detailed knowledge of various physiologic patterns associated with one or more stages of sleep. An attempt was made to develop detectors or indicators that highlight specific EEG patterns such as "K-complexes," "sleep spindles," or "delta waveforms" which sleep researchers find meaningful. Additional information was extracted from two EOG channels to determine the occurrence of REM and to assist in classifying REM sleep.

II. DATA PROCESSING

The data used for designing and evaluating the classification systems were provided by NMNPRU.[1] As part of a study concerning the effects of sleep deprivation, over 30 young adult male subjects, ages 17 to 21, were recorded during presleep waking and during all-night sleep. No medication was used to induce sleep. At least one channel of EEG was recorded from the central (top) position of the head and referred to a mastoid electrode located behind the subject's ear. Two channels of horizontal EOG's were obtained from electrodes attached to the outer canthus of each eye (in the crow's feet) to monitor eye movements. An electronic time code signal was also recorded to provide cross reference between the chart recordings read by the human sleep scorer and the data processed by computer. The sleep records were scored manually by NMNPRU using criteria specified in the Standard Sleep Scoring Manual (Rechtschaffen and Kales, 1968) produced by the Association for the Psychophysiological Study of Sleep (APSS). The overnight recordings ranged from $5\frac{1}{2}$ to 8 hr in length.

Computer processing of the recorded data was accomplished as illustrated in Fig. 2: (1) analog-to-digital conversion; (2) spectral analysis of EEG; (3) measurement of delta activity; (4) pattern recognition of EEG (decision tree); (5) REM detection and scoring logic program

A. A/D Conversion

The analog information was converted to digital form at an effective sampling rate of 68.3 samples per second per channel. A 5-min period of 10 Hz sine wave, 100 μV amplitude, served as the calibration signal. Subsequent computer programs scaled all data values to conform to this standard. Timing signals were decoded and merged with the digital data. EEG was filtered to attenuate frequencies above 28 Hz. The EOG was filtered to attenuate frequencies above 14 Hz. Higher sampling rates and frequency response were used during the investigative phase of the program. The final sampling rate was a compromise involving a trade-off between volume of stored data and the usefulness of higher frequency information.

---

[1] The Navy Medical Neuropsychiatric Research Unit, San Diego, Calif. under the direction of Dr. L. C. Johnson conducted the sleep research which provided the data used for the pattern recognition studies. In addition, Dr. Johnson and his colleagues manually scored many overnight records for the system performance evaluation. Their assistance and support is greatly appreciated.

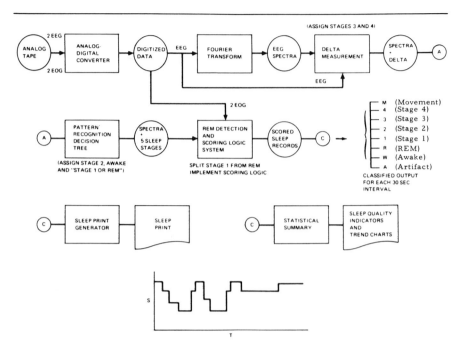

FIG. 2. Automatic sleep scoring system.

B. Spectral Analysis of EEG

The second step consisted of performing a Fourier analysis of successive 30-sec epochs of EEG. Figure 3 is a computer-generated plot showing both the original EEG and the Fourier amplitude spectrum for that epoch. Since many of the patterns used for identifying sleep states are rhythmic and quasi-sinusoidal, the Fourier transform provided a means for extracting this frequency information. Initial experiments used fine frequency resolution with a separate spectral indicator for each successive 0.2-Hz band. Later results showed no notable loss in performance when frequency resolution was reduced to provide one indicator for each 1-Hz increment up to 34 Hz. (The DC component was ignored since the original data were AC-coupled.) The 34 spectral intensity values were stored on digital tape for analysis by the pattern recognition system.

C. Measurement of Delta Activity

Attempts to match human discrimination between Stages 3 and 4 using Fourier analysis were of marginal success. The Fourier transform measured

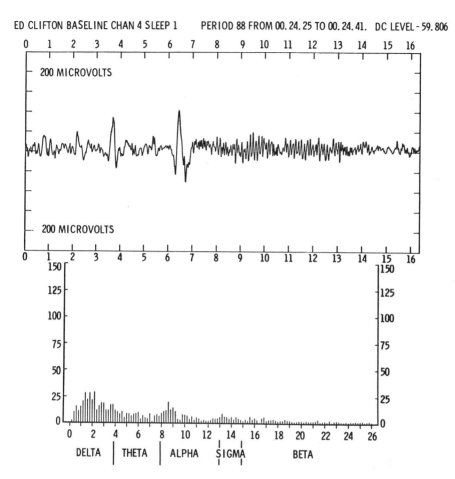

ED CLIFTON BASELINE CHAN 4 SLEEP 1   PERIOD 88 FROM 00. 24. 25 TO 00. 24. 41. DC LEVEL - 59. 806

FIG. 3. Analog signal with resulting spectrum.

the amount of energy in the delta frequency band (0 to 2 Hz). However, it was found that the human scorer's technique of counting the number of low-frequency waves ($\leq$ 2 Hz) which exceeded 75 μV produced results which were not proportional to the energy in the band from 0 to 2 Hz. Therefore, the pattern recognition procedure described in the next section was unable to produce acceptable matching of the human classification of Stages 3 and 4. This led to development of a substitute computer program employing known property extraction techniques to determine the amount of delta activity in a manner similar to that used by human scorers.

The delta measurement program examined successive 30-sec increments of EEG data to locate peaks no closer than 0.5 sec, corresponding to activity of 2 Hz or less. The program accepted as delta activity those portions of the record in which the peak-to-valley difference exceeded 75 μV and which had at least a 0.75 correlation coefficient with a straight line drawn between the peak and valley. Stage 3 and Stage 4 classifications are assigned on the basis of percentage of the epoch involved in delta activity. A provision for a slight relaxation of the delta percentage criterion after the subject had entered Stage 4 provided closer agreement with human scorers.

D. Pattern Recognition of EEG

If, for a particular 30-sec epoch, a Stage 3 or Stage 4 classification had not been assigned by the delta measurement program, the epoch's frequency pattern consisting of 34 spectral indicators was presented to a decision tree. This tree or classification network was composed of two separate pattern recognition systems.

The structure of the basic pattern recognition system (Fig. 4) consists of two layers of active components — property filters and the response unit. The property filters operate on a limited subset of the input data, typically six of the 34 possible input connections. The property filters attempt to extract clues concerning pattern identity from the input patterns. The outputs of the property filters are weighted and summed in the response unit which assigns the pattern to one of two classes. The design of the pattern recognition system involves a learning algorithm applied to EEG records divided into 30-sec intervals and previously manually scored into one of the remaining sleep states.

The pattern recognition learning algorithm used in this study is called the "discriminant-analysis, iterative-design" (DAID) technique (Viglione, 1970). It uses two levels of decision as indicated in Fig. 4. The input to the system is the array (or vector) of numbers representing the energy in the different frequency bands.

Each of the first level decisions use only six of the values of the vector as the basis for its decision. The mean and covariance matrix for this vector are estimated from the preclassified samples[2] for the appropriate sleep state. Then the coefficients and threshold are calculated that would best differentiate two Gaussian distributions with these mean vectors and covariance matrices. A quadratic function of these six values is calculated for each EEG sample, and a "zero" or "one" output is generated as the function value does or does not exceed a threshold:

---

[2] Preclassified samples refer to the set of EEG data that has been labeled by manual interpretation methods as to the state of sleep of the subject on an epoch (30-sec) by epoch basis. This is also referred to as the design set of data.

$$f\underset{=}{\Delta} \sum_{i=1}^{6} a_i v_i + \sum_{i=1}^{6} \sum_{j=1}^{6} b_{ij} v_i v_j \begin{cases} > \Theta \text{ property filter output equals 1} \\ < \Theta \text{ property filter output equals 0} \end{cases}$$

where the v_i are the values for each frequency band and the a_i, b_i, and Θ are the derived terms for the discriminant function.

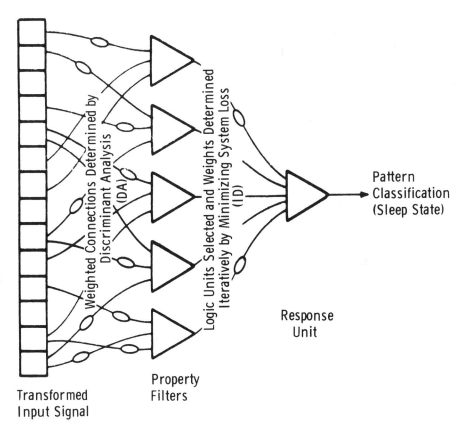

FIG. 4. Pattern recognition system.

The one-zero decision of the candidate preliminary decision units would be well correlated with the identification of two different sleep states, if the selected spectral energy components were distributed according to different multivariate Gaussian distributions. Unfortunately this is improbable. Most likely, however, there is some correlation, and the one/zero decision of the first layer candidate does carry significant information. The task of the learning algorithm is to incorporate this information into the second level decision in an optimum manner.

The second level decision element (response unit) is chosen to be a linear decision; that is, a linear function of the numerical values of the first layer decisions is calculated, and a one or zero decision is made dependent on whether this does or does not exceed a threshold:

$$g \triangleq \sum c_i \gamma_i \begin{cases} > \varphi \text{ assign the pattern to class 1} \\ < \varphi \text{ assign the pattern to class 0} \end{cases}$$

where the γ_i are the first-layer decision variables and φ is the threshold of the second-layer decision element.

The coefficients c_i and the particular candidate property filters or first-layer units to be incorporated in the second-layer decision process are determined by the "iterative design" technique. This technique is characterized by three criteria: (1) the definition of an optimization criterion, called a loss function; (2) the determination of the coefficient c_i for each candidate logic unit that would best improve the loss function; (3) the selection of those units from the candidate population which, with their optimal coefficients, most reduce the loss.

The loss function depends again on the use of the preclassified sample of patterns. For each pattern, j, a value L_j is defined

$$L_j = e^{-\delta_j(g_j - \varphi)}$$

where L_j is called the loss associated with sample j

$$\delta_j = \begin{cases} -1 \text{ if sample } j \text{ is in class 1} \\ 1 \text{ if sample } j \text{ is in class 0} \end{cases}$$

The total loss L is then:

$$L = \sum_{j=1}^{N} L_j = \sum_{j=1}^{N} e^{-\delta_j(g_j - \varphi)}$$

The values of c_i and φ which optimize this function are then derived through a cyclic relaxation process (hence, the use of the "iterative" term in the design acronym) where each pattern in the design set is examined and its contribution evaluated.

Two separate classification systems are designed. The first separates Stage 2 epochs from Awake, Stage 1, and REM. The second separates Awake from the Stage 1/REM epochs.

E. REM Detection and Logic Program

The REM-LOGIC Program represented the last step in the classification process. The spectral indicators were processed to determine the presence of movement or artifact. If the classification "Stage 1 or REM" had been assigned by the pattern recognition decision tree, the raw digital tape was searched for conjugate REM, on the two EOG channels. If no eye movements were found, the sleep record was "scanned" both forward and back to determine activity before and after the low-voltage, mixed-frequency periods. Great care was exercised in designing this scoring logic to match the actions and decisions of the human scorer and to incorporate criteria expressed in the standard scoring manual. For example, a stretch of "Stage 1 or REM" activity preceded and followed by Stage 2 epochs was classified as Stage 1 if longer than 3 min; otherwise, the intervening low-voltage activity was scored as Stage 2. Evaluation and feedback by experienced sleep scorers led to numerous refinements to this program and incorporation of additional logic decisions.

In addition, the frequency indicators are also processed to detect the presence of gross body movements, contaminating noise, and spurious artifacts. Body movement and artifact detection are both based on the thresholding of the power contained in the higher frequencies.

The corresponding output from this REM detection and logic operation is used to supplement or override the classification of the pattern recognition systems. A movement detection will override all classifications other than Stages 3 and 4. A REM detection will override the Stage 1 classification, and a Stage 2 classification if that epoch is preceded by a movement; finally, the artifact detection will override all decision tree classifications and cause the last epoch classification to be carried through until the artifact is over. Figure 5 is an example of the computer printout illustrating the operation of the automatic scoring system.

The output from the scoring system was finally processed by a computer program from which the sleep print was generated. Four adjacent 30-sec classification outputs were averaged and a sleep stage noted for that 2-min interval. Each 2-min interval was plotted to provide a ready display of the subject's sleep over the entire sleep period as illustrated previously in Fig. 1. In addition, the quantities used to evaluate the quality of the subject's sleep were also computed. These 45 parameters include length of time in each stage, total sleep time, total awake time, number of movements, and number of sleep transitions, among others (see Fig. 6). The entire operation, digitizing, frequency analysis, . . . , through sleep scoring and statistical

Time	Scoring System Output		REM Logic and Artifact Detector Output	Manual Scoring	
03:34:00	STAGE	2		STAGE	2
03:34:30	STAGE	2		STAGE	2
03:35:00	STAGE	2		STAGE	2
03:35:30	STAGE	2		STAGE	2
03:36:00	STAGE	2		STAGE	2
03:36:30	STAGE	2		STAGE	2
03:37:00	STAGE	2		ARTIFACT	
03:37:30	STAGE	2		ARTIFACT	
03:38:00	STAGE	2		STAGE	2
03:38:30	STAGE	2		STAGE	2
03:39:00	AWAKE			ARTIFACT	
03:39:30	STAGE ·	2		ARTIFACT	
03:40:00	STAGE	2		STAGE	2
03:40:30	STAGE	2		STAGE	2
03:41:00	STAGE	2		STAGE	2
03:41:30	STAGE	2		STAGE	2
03:42:00	STAGE	2		STAGE	2
03:42:30	STAGE	2		STAGE	2
03:43:00	STAGE	2		STAGE	2
03:43:30	AWAKE			STAGE	2
03:44:00	REM		REM	TRANSIT.	
03:44:30	REM		REM	REM	
03:45:00	REM			REM	
03:45:30	REM		ARTIFACT	ARTIFACT	
03:46:00	REM		ARTIFACT	ARTIFACT	
03:46:30	REM		ARTIFACT	ARTIFACT	
03:47:00	REM		ARTIFACT	ARTIFACT	
03:47:30	REM		ARTIFACT	ARTIFACT	
03:48:00	REM		ARTIFACT	ARTIFACT	
03:48:30	REM		REM	ARTIFACT	
03:49:00	REM			ARTIFACT	
03:49:30	REM		REM	ARTIFACT	
03:50:00	REM		ARTIFACT	MOVEMENT	
03:50:30	REM			MOVEMENT	
03:51:00	REM			REM	
03:51:30	REM			REM	
03:52:00	REM			REM	
03:52:30	REM			REM	
03:53:00	REM			REM	
03:53:30	REM		REM	REM	
03:54:00	REM		REM	REM	
03:54:30	REM			REM	
03:55:00	REM		REM	REM	

FIG. 5. Automatic sleep scoring, computer printout.

Sleep Parameters

#	Parameter	Value	Unit
1	TOTAL BED TIME	488	MINUTES
2	TOTAL SLEEP TIME	480	MINUTES
3	TOTAL WAKE TIME	64	MINUTES
4	TOTAL STAGE 1	202	MINUTES
5	TOTAL STAGE 2	46	MINUTES
6	TOTAL STAGE 3	84	MINUTES
7	TOTAL STAGE 4	84	MINUTES
8	TOTAL STAGE REM	24	MINUTES
9	TOTAL STAGE NON-REM	396	MINUTES
10	TOTAL MOVEMENT TIME	130	MINUTES
11	TOTAL STAGE NON-REM	332	MINUTES
12	TOTAL OF STAGES 3 AND 4	4	MINUTES
13	TOTAL OF STAGES 2, 3, AND 4	0	MINUTES
14	WAKE TIME BEFORE THE FIRST STAGE 2	0	MINUTES
15	WAKE TIME DURING SLEEP	12	MINUTES
16	WAKE TIME AFTER LAST SLEEP	122	MINUTES
17	TIME BEFORE THE FIRST STAGE 2	204	MINUTES
18	TIME BEFORE THE FIRST STAGE 3		MINUTES
19	TIME BEFORE THE FIRST STAGE 4		MINUTES
20	TIME BEFORE THE FIRST STAGE REM		MINUTES
21	AVERAGE DURATION OF MOVEMENTS	.8	MINUTES
22	AVERAGE DURATION OF AROUSALS	4.2	MINUTES
23	AVERAGE DURATION OF STAGE NON-REM	100.2	MINUTES
24	AVERAGE DURATION OF STAGE REM	29.3	MINUTES
25	AVERAGE REM-TO-REM INTERVAL	84.2	MINUTES
26	PERCENT WAKE OF TOTAL BED TIME	.82	PERCENT
27	PERCENT SLEEP OF TOTAL BED TIME	98.36	PERCENT
28	PERCENT MOVEMENT TIME OF TOTAL BED TIME	4.82	PERCENT
29	PERCENT WAKE BEFORE FIRST STAGE 2 OF TOTAL WAKE TIME	100.00	PERCENT
30	PERCENT OF WAKE DURING SLEEP OF TOTAL WAKE TIME	.00	PERCENT
31	PERCENT OF WAKE AFTER SLEEP TO TOTAL WAKE TIME	13.33	PERCENT
32	PERCENT STAGE 1 OF TOTAL SLEEP TIME	42.08	PERCENT
33	PERCENT STAGE 2 OF TOTAL SLEEP TIME	9.58	PERCENT
34	PERCENT STAGE 3 OF TOTAL SLEEP TIME	17.50	PERCENT
35	PERCENT STAGE 4 OF TOTAL SLEEP TIME	17.50	PERCENT
36	PERCENT STAGE REM OF TOTAL SLEEP TIME	82.50	PERCENT
37	PERCENT STAGE NON-REM OF TOTAL SLEEP TIME	27.08	PERCENT
38	PERCENT STAGES 3 AND 4 OF TOTAL SLEEP TIME	69.17	PERCENT
39	PERCENT STAGES 2, 3, AND 4 OF TOTAL SLEEP TIME	28	PERCENT
40	NUMBER OF MOVEMENT EPISODES	7	
41	NUMBER OF AROUSAL EPISODES	4	
42	NUMBER OF STAGE NON-REM EPISODES	3	
43	NUMBER OF STAGE REM EPISODES		
44	NUMBER OF STAGE CHANGES	44	
45	DISTRIBUTION OF EPISODE DURATION IN MINUTES		

```
MOVEMENT   27 4 6 8 10 12 14 16 18 20 22 24 26 28 30 32 34 36 38 40 42 44 46 48 50 52 54 56 58 60 62 64 66 68 70 72 74 76 78 1HI
AROUSAL     5
NON-REM     5
REM
45. TIME OF EACH REM-TO-REM INTERVAL IN MINUTES
    97.5  71.0
```

FIG. 6. Sleep parameters.

summary and plotting, requires approximately 3 to $3\frac{1}{2}$ hr for each 9- to 10-hr sleep period using the XDS-930 computer.

III. SYSTEM VALIDATION

To test the validity of the results of the automatic sleep scoring system, an experiment was designed using overnight sleep recordings from nine subjects. Data from four of the subjects provided the design or training set. After the automatic scoring system had been designed and "tuned" on the original four subjects, all design parameters and thresholds were frozen and the system was tested on overnight sleep records from five independent subjects. Each recording was obtained on the fourth laboratory night of sleep. The Offner chart recordings corresponding to the five test records were classified independently by three experienced human scorers.[3] These judges took extra care to follow the criteria set forth in the Standard Scoring Manual for determining stages of sleep.

Table 1 summarizes the results of the study. Three percentages are shown for each of the five subjects included in the study. The first column is the average pairwise agreement for the human scorers. This figure was obtained by computing the percent agreement between judges 1 and 2, judges 2 and 3, and judges 1 and 3. These three figures were averaged for each subject. The second column represents the average of the three percent agreements obtained between the computer and each of the three judges. The third column is the percent agreement between the computer and the consensus scoring produced by the majority of three judges.

TABLE 1. Summary of percent agreement for five subjects, all stages of sleep (stages 1–4, awake, and REM)

Subject	Average percent agreement of judge vs. judge	Average percent agreement of computer vs. judge	Percent agreement of computer vs. consensus
02	91.4	86.2	86.3
06	87.8	77.7	79.3
11	85.8	77.7	78.8
12	90.9	78.7	79.6
13	90.8	83.5	86.4
Overall average	89.3	80.8	82.1

[3]The judges are qualified sleep researchers with lengthy experience in human performance monitoring and analysis of EEG for sleep scoring.

In every case the average percent agreement between two judges was higher than between computer and consensus. The difference between the first and third columns of Table 1 ranged from 4.4% for subject 13 to 11.3% for subject 12. For every subject, average pairwise agreement between the computer and individual judges was slightly lower than for computer versus consensus, supporting the assumption that the consensus judgment is "better," or at least more stable, than that of an individual scorer.

Stages 3 and 4 are defined to represent degrees of slow-wave sleep. For some studies this distinction is not required, and Stages 3 and 4 may be combined into a single stage referred to as slow-wave sleep. Table 2 presents a summary of the agreement study results under the assumption that five sleep stages are scored (Awake, REM, Stage 1, Stage 2, and Slow-Wave Sleep) with criteria for determining the transition from Stage 2 to slow-wave sleep remaining the same as for the transition to Stage 3. All classes of agreement show an increase, but the difference between judge versus judge and computer versus consensus has dropped to 6.4%.

TABLE 2. Summary of percent agreement for five subjects, one stage for slow-wave sleep (stages 3 and 4 combined)

Subject	Average percent agreement of judge vs. judge	Average percent agreement of computer vs. judge	Percent agreement of computer vs. consensus
02	92.6	88.0	88.6
06	89.3	80.4	81.6
11	89.8	82.2	83.3
12	92.3	81.6	82.6
13	92.7	86.7	88.6
Overall average	91.3	83.9	84.9

As a final comparison, percent agreement on a stage-by-stage basis was performed over all subjects for judge versus judge and computer versus consensus. The results are displayed in Table 3. For the three categories in which computer performance was lowest, humans also exhibited poor agreement.

The computer's identification of Awake periods was unsatisfactory. Examination of the chart recordings showed little alpha activity on the central EEG channel used by the computer and indicated the human scorers had utilized secondary information provided by another EEG channel and other data, particularly time of night, to assist in their scoring.

TABLE 3. Percent agreement stage-by-stage, averaged overall five subjects

Scorers	Sleep stage					
	Awake	Stage 1	REM	Stage 2	Stage 3	Stage 4
Judge vs. judge	67.8	60.5	93.4	93.0	60.3	80.3
Computer vs. consensus	3.0	61.6	86.6	87.7	59.8	91.5

The computer's percent agreement with the consensus on Stage 1 and Stage 3 was virtually identical with the agreement among experienced human scorers.

In the past, sleep scorers evaluating automatic scoring systems have indicated that 50 to 60% agreement on Stage 3 was not satisfactory. However, Table 3 demonstrates that the computer shows the same percent agreement with the consensus of human judges as those same judges show among themselves. These results imply that the delta measurement techniques employed by the automatic sleep scoring system are at least as reliable as the human visual analysis. The reliability between human scorers for Stage 3 sets the upper limit for the reliability between the computer and human scorers, even if the computer correctly classified all Stage epochs according to the APSS manual. These results support the arguments of those who consider Stage 3 as a transitional stage and would lump Stages 3 and 4 into a single slow-wave sleep stage.

IV. CONCLUSIONS

The computer scoring system reported in this paper has undergone numerous changes in response to evaluation by pattern recognition specialists and sleep scorers. The original approach employed pattern recognition techniques applied to the Fourier spectrum of one channel of EEG in discriminating all stages of sleep. This approach reflected the desires expressed by some sleep researchers for scoring sleep by monitoring a minimum number of physiologic parameters. It was subsequently shown that no reliable means of distinguishing between Stage 1 and REM could be found based only on frequency analysis of one EEG channel (Martin, Viglione, Johnson, and Naitoh, 1971).

As a result, the system was expanded to include techniques for detecting and identifying conjugate eye movements from two horizontal EOG channels. In addition, it was apparent that a system which scored the EEG by looking only at the epoch under consideration could not possibly match the human who scanned forward and backward through the record before making decisions. This observation led to insertion of logic to match the human decision-making process upon preceding and following stage transitions, particularly for runs of Stage 1 epochs.

It also became clear that techniques using analog filtering, digital spectral analysis, or period analysis were subject to failure in matching human discrimination between Stages 3 and 4 (and possibly 2). These techniques basically reflect the low-frequency energy present in the EEG trace. The visual scoring criteria are *not* proportional to low-frequency energy because of the 75-μV threshold required for acceptance as delta activity. The delta measurement technique was substituted for the spectral analysis in the determination of delta to achieve closer agreement with human scorers. This does not mean that spectral analysis or analog filtering of delta activity should be abandoned. It is believed that spectral analysis provides a more sensitive and reliable tool for examining nocturnal delta EEG activity. For example, Fig. 7 shows a profile of low-frequency EEG activity during sleep. This profile illustrates clearly the cyclic nature of delta activity which occurs throughout the night. This delta cycle is usually not detected by visual scoring, since these early morning periods do not normally reach the Stage 3 criterion and the human bias is to score early morning delta sleep as Stage 2.

Recent investigations have shown that scoring of transitional epochs is highly sensitive to a 10% error in determining the 75-μV threshold. If future

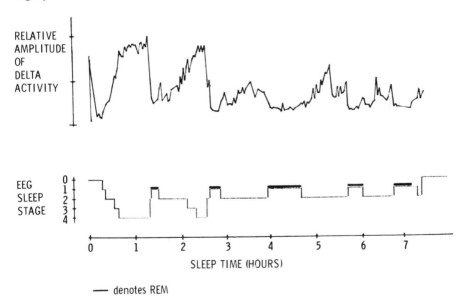

FIG. 7. Delta activity (0.2 to 2 Hz) and sleep stages vs. sleep time (Subject 02S baseline).

standards for measurement of slow-wave activity were based upon spectral intensity criteria rather than the present visual criteria, a more reliable and sensitive indicator of changes in slow-wave with age, drugs, or illness might be possible.

This study reports an approach to using a pattern recognition system, simulated on a digital computer, for automatic, all-night sleep scoring. Based upon a detailed comparison of percent agreement for the computer and three experienced human judges, the computer scoring system has achieved a satisfactory performance level and may be considered as a useful alternative to visual sleep stage scoring. Performance is expected to increase with provision of a more reliable means of identifying awake periods. In addition, the system design can be readily modified to accommodate specific subjects with the attendant increase in classification accuracy.

The techniques used in the development of this system also have applicability to the general problem of automating the processing and analysis of the electroencephalographic, and other, physiologic parameters. This should provide an adjunct to the routine and clinical monitoring and assessment of human performance, physical condition, susceptibility to physical and psychologic stress and general clinical diagnosis.

V. SUMMARY

Historically, sleep staging has involved the manual editing and analysis of hours of EEG and EOG data by qualified encephalographers. To alleviate this tedious and time-consuming task and to eliminate the inherent subjective nature of manual interpretation, an automatic method for processing this EEG/EOG data has been developed using advanced techniques of pattern recognition and computer processing. The various analytic procedures investigated are discussed, illustrating the problems involved in attempting to emulate human analysts. Performance of the final system is evaluated against that of three qualified sleep researchers.

ACKNOWLEDGMENT

This work was sponsored in part by the Physiologic Psychology Branch of the Office of Naval Research.

REFERENCES

Dement, W., and Kleitman, N. (1957): Cyclic variations in EEG during sleep and their relation to eye movements, body motility, and dreaming. *Electroencephalography and Clinical Neurophysiology,* 9:673–689.

Martin, W. B., Viglione, S. S., Johnson, L. C., and Naitoh, P. (1971): Pattern recognition of EEG to determine level of alertness. *Electroencephalography and Clinical Neurophysiology,* 30:163.

Rechtschaffen, A., and Kales, A. (1968): *Manual of Standardized Terminology, Techniques, and Scoring System for Sleep Stages of Human Subjects.* National Institutes of Health Publication No. 204, U.S. Government Printing Office, Washington, D.C. 57 pp.

Viglione, S. S. (1970): Applications of pattern recognition technology. In: *Adaptive, Learning, and Pattern Recognition System Theory and Applications,* edited by J. M. Mendel and K. S. Fu. Academic Press, New York, pp. 115–162.

Automation of Clinical Electroencephalography.
Edited by P. Kellaway and I. Petersén.
Raven Press, New York © 1973.

Comments on Pattern Recognition*

S. S. Viglione

Research and Development Directorate, McDonnell Douglas Astronautics Company, Huntington Beach, California 92647

Almost every contributor to this volume addresses himself to the problem of pattern recognition. I have been active in this field for about 15 years, and no one has yet told me much about pattern recognition. Many have used the term and have alluded to the concept in articles and talks, but I question whether we in fact have a common understanding of what is meant by the term "pattern recognition." I will attempt in this chapter to categorize what I see as pattern recognition and perhaps place what is included in this volume in that context, thereby providing a common framework that readily identifies the various facets of a pattern recognition design and highlights those areas which hold the most promise for automation and aided analysis of the EEG.

Methodology is generally illustrated via a very simple block diagram that shows what processes occur in a pattern recognition design (Fig. 1). Here the term "preprocessing" implies that you take some sensory information at the input (we are concerned with the EEG) and perform an operation to condition that EEG. The preprocessing may take on a simple form, perhaps only an amplification or an analog-to-digital conversion or a bandpass filtering of some kind. This has little to do with the identification of the epoch or event in the EEG. Perhaps the preprocessing attempts to increase the S/N ratio of the epoch, but that is about all. Or perhaps it puts the data into a more convenient format for subsequent analysis.

---

*This chapter is an edited version of an extemporaneous discourse by the author at the Conference on Automation in Clinical Electroencephalography.

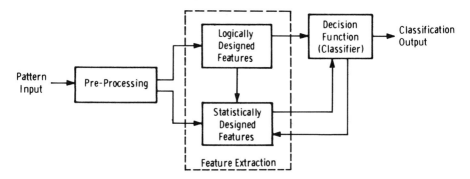

FIG. 1. Pattern recognition mechanism.

The second step (Fig. 1) involves a detailed look at the data, either the preprocessed or raw data. That is usually called the extraction of information, features, or properties. This is known as "feature extraction," and it can take on many different forms. The data can be examined subjectively, and it is determined that information regarding the spikeness of the pattern is to be extracted. Or, alternatively, perhaps the interest is in the delta or slow-wave activity, and methods for extracting information on the energy in the low-frequency bands is sought. These are features that one can extract either from the raw or conditioned data. I would contend that most of the discussions we have had on pattern recognition have centered on methods for doing feature extraction. The taking of first and second derivatives of the data, and their threshold, as well as methods for examining the waveforms and trying to define an identifier so that at a later time the waveform can be coded, have been discussed

In pattern recognition design, we go one step further. Based on this feature set, we attempt to obtain a decision about the state of the EEG. We derive a decision function (Fig. 1). The problem of deriving this decision function, *per se,* is not discussed in this volume. Perhaps if the second derivative information were extracted, a threshold specified, and a rule established that if the signal is above the threshold, then the decision is made that a spike occurred; surely that may be a decision function, albeit a simple one. The matched filter is another example of a method of pattern recognition. In matched filtering, selected information — a feature — is extracted. Then a decision function is performed by correlating that filter with the signal and determining if that correlation exceeds a certain value, a threshold occurs. If it does, then it is noted that the signal feature was present. In that sense, some of the ingredients of pattern recognition are used in applying matched filtering and thresholding. In reality, however, we have never used the depth of processing that is available when you look at the mechanism of pattern recognition as an entity, of designing a decision function to influence how features and perhaps even the preprocessing are designed. The design of a pattern recognition system should consider all these facets in concert. The recognition system design does not entail just one part, but the entity; this is the position I take in my discussion of pattern recognition.

In the context of EEG analysis and the previous discussions, how does one design a decision function? Here the analytic processes of adaptive or learning theory become involved. How does one specify features? Many methods have been discussed for specifying features for EEG. How does one correlate these features? It is the task of the decision function to relate these features to the events and the events themselves to a classification. If we use this design philosophy, we also have available to us some way of attacking the problem that Dr. Kellaway addressed. Suppose that as you are looking at an electroencephalograph you have this visceral feeling that something is changing in the record. Later you see the occurrence of the spike events in the pattern. How do you convey this information, this feeling that you had that the record was changing? By working within the framework of the pattern recognition design discussed, it may suffice only to note that "there's something different in this record." As the record progresses, a change can be verified and some meaning attached to it. For design purposes a note is made at this point in the record, "I have a suspicion that something is changing. I can't identify it, but here's the record. Can you search the record to find out if there are any differences in this time interval where I only had a suspicion (or may not have even felt) that there were changes occurring, as opposed to this period where I can definitely show the spikiness of the pattern? Is there something in here?" If an attempt at feature extraction is made, as some suggest, it would be difficult because there are no real indications to guide you. But, in fact, one can digitize this data, and from the raw digital data try to extract information using the framework of the pattern recognition design. This is the approach we have taken in the design of our pattern recognition work.

Let me suggest a method that can be used to design a decision function that has a secondary purpose of being able to evaluate features. I will address myself to designing a classifier and use a procedure that will also help define what are the best features to be used for the specific problem. A simple model will suffice for demonstration. Let me use a threshold logic unit.

This threshold logic unit (see Fig. 2) is defined in terms of function $\sum_i b_i w_i$ and a threshold θ, a variable. I proceed with the assumption that a number of indicators, i.e., features, have been extracted as illustrated in Fig. 3. I will just list these features. I do not know what they signify, and it is of little importance. We intend to develop a system whereby the effectiveness of these features can be evaluated. The output from each one of these features, e.g., $b_1 \ldots b_n$, is taken, and a variable weighting function $(w_i \ldots w_n)$ is applied to each. A variable threshold is also a design specification. This

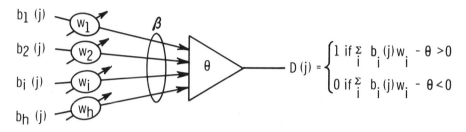

$$D(j) = \begin{cases} 1 \text{ if } \sum_i b_i(j)w_i - \theta > 0 \\ 0 \text{ if } \sum_i b_i(j)w_i - \theta < 0 \end{cases}$$

FIG. 2. Threshold logic unit.

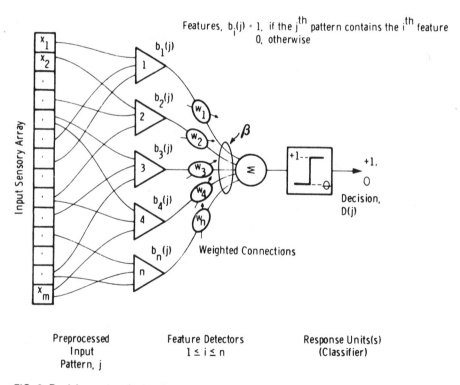

Features, $b_i(j) = 1$, if the jth pattern contains the ith feature
0, otherwise

Preprocessed
Input
Pattern, j

Feature Detectors
$1 \leq i \leq n$

Response Units(s)
(Classifier)

FIG. 3. Decision network structure.

threshold logic will be considered to have only one of two states (either high or low) and one of a two-class problem (spike or no-spike).

Having established this model, we can derive a method for organizing it which would adaptively derive these weighting functions, specifying the threshold and maybe even selecting the features. To do this, several ground rules must be established. A set of data must be selected that contains examples of both types of pattern, i.e., spike and no-spike. Then a mathematical function is defined to represent the input to the threshold logic unit. This function, β in Figs. 2 and 3, is equal to the sum of each feature output times its weight $\beta = \sum_i b_i w_i$. The threshold logic unit compares this summation to a threshold. When an input signal is applied and this sum is greater than the threshold, then the signal (or pattern) belongs to the positive class (spikes), and if it is less than the threshold, it belongs to the negative class (no-spikes). We will work with this term $\beta - \theta$, taking the exponential form of this term exp $(\beta - \theta)$, and multiplying it by a pattern factor δ, which is $+1$ for a known spike pattern and -1 for a non-spike pattern. This δ is solely a means for identifying the data input during the design phase. For each of these data patterns that make up the design set, a "loss" number is assigned, the loss of the j-th pattern, $L_j = \exp - \delta(\beta - \theta)$. A controlling design is defined which guarantees that this structure will converge to a set of weights and thresholds capable of separating patterns in the design set. The design function is a system loss, which is merely the sum of these pattern losses over all the patterns, $SL = \sum_j L_j$. Then the controlling design criterion is the minimization of the system loss. Available to achieve this minimization are the weights and the threshold. Every time I input a data point, if the pattern is correctly classified, the exponential term should be negative. As a result, this loss number should be small. However, if the pattern is incorrectly classified, the converse is true: the exponent is positive and the loss number will be large. Correctly classified patterns give rise to small loss numbers and have little influence on the total system loss. Incorrectly classified patterns exert a large impact on the system loss. The weights of the features and of the threshold are modified to reduce the system loss for each pattern.

One other variable is the indicator "i." It refers to the feature that I have extracted. Assume one wants to evaluate the effectiveness of a candidate set of features. One feature at a time, for example, can be introduced, and its effect in minimizing this system loss determined. If a reduction in system loss is not achieved, the feature can be discarded and another attempt made. Of course, each time this is done the weights and the threshold should be readjusted.

This is just one method of recognition system design. We have good techniques for designing these decision functions. This is not the major problem area. Generally when investigators address themselves to the problem of feature extraction, which I suspect most do, they actually are concerned with the heart of pattern recognition. However, the design discussed allows for determination of the effectiveness of the features by examination of the appropriate weights. The decision function is the guide in the design of the feature extraction. The choice of the exponential form of the decision function satisfies two requirements: a monotonic decreasing function that would converge and a good criterion to measure how well the system is performing. If we consider the number of errors the system is making on a sample of the data versus the number of features added, the error rate describes a system performance curve. The exponential form of the system loss follows this error curve very nicely. It therefore provides a good indication of how well the system works in terms of classification performance.

GENERAL DISCUSSION

Dumermuth expressed pessimism about the possibility of achieving comprehensive and economical automation of clinical EEG with resources that are available at the present time. First, the technological problem of acquiring and analyzing complicated multi-channel information from several recordings simultaneously are enormous. Also, there are likely to be major problems in finding the highly skilled and specialized personnel who would be needed to operate an automated EEG system. Frost replied that he recognized these problems and agreed that a fully automated EEG laboratory was still several years away. However, in his view, the way to tackle the problem was to introduce automatic data processing gradually into the operational frame of reference that he had outlined. Thus one had to look at an automatic EEG system as one that could grow slowly rather than one that could be put into operation forthwith, using existing technology. Maulsby did not share Dumermuth's pessimism about the possibility of achieving an economically viable automatic EEG system. He considered that Frost had performed a useful service in departmentalizing the different sorts of disciplines and areas that people would have to work on in a project of this kind. Frost's analysis of the problem permitted decisions about the personnel that would be required to work on each block in the project diagram and allowed practical decisions to be made about the kind of funding that will be required. Levy commented that he realized that each component of the overall problem defined by Frost had not been solved completely and that such solutions would involve creative intellectual work of the highest order. However, it was apparent that most of the participants at the conference felt that they could, given the resources, tackle finite pieces of the problem with a high probability of success, and that such partial solutions could eventually be put together into a comprehensive system. On the basis of the contributions that he had heard, Levy felt that this confidence was justified. One matter in which Levy was particularly interested was the role of larger computers in an automated EEG system. Nobody had any doubts about the usefulness of hybrid and special-purpose devices, and the remaining question was whether there was indeed any role at all for larger computers. At the present time he thought that they would probably interact with the EEG laboratory via a terminal, and that the larger computer, apart from its potential value as a data bank, could be regarded as something of a switching device to enable acquisition and processing of information from other laboratories, possibly in other centers, thus enlarging the data base from which diagnostic decisions could be elaborated. Kaiser reemphasized the necessity for including sensors and analysis procedures for detecting and evaluating spurious signals that might be due to such factors as muscle activity, movement, and changes in the electrodes.

Automation of Clinical Electroencephalography.
Edited by P. Kellaway and I. Petersén.
Raven Press, New York © 1973.

Two Classes of Feature-Extracting Processes

Donald O. Walter

Faculty of Medicine, Marseille, France, and Brain Research Institute, U.C.L.A., Los Angeles, California

Computation-heavy processes such as digital spectral analysis, auto-correlation analysis, or digital matched filtering compensate for the lengthy machine time they require by being sensitive to small or obscured features in data, such as small waves or small harmonics of waves. Averaging evoked potentials has a similar property, although its computation time is not great and is masked by the data acquisition or access time. I seem to consider in this class those methods derived or derivable from linear theory. Such methods respond also to large, dominant waves, giving indications which can be related sensibly to the indications they give about the smaller or hidden waves. However, there are some parameters which cannot at all, or not very easily, be estimated by these methods, usually because the parameters are not clearly definable for obscured waves.

On the other hand, there are processes, generally computation-light, such as zero crossing, phase-locked loops, and extremum detection, which have contrasting sensitivities: they respond poorly to small or hidden waves, but they give indications concerning large, dominant waves which are easily understood and related to the visually obvious properties of such waves. These methods have existed in EEG analysis for some time, but in a somewhat inhibited form, because their users usually did not know their theoretical properties — indeed, often no one knew them, since they are essentially nonlinear in their mathematical description. In the last few years, however, versions of such methods have been reported in the engineering literature,

295

and the theory of stochastic processes, or some related theory, has been used to shed some theoretical light on the properties of these methods.

At the moment, there seems to be the potential for great argument between proponents of the two classes of methods (see, for example, Reports of the 1st APSS International Meeting, edited by M. Chase et al.; section on Computers edited by L. C. Johnson). I hope these disagreements can be reduced by presenting the two classes of methods within a common conspectus, from which applications can be designed for cost-effectiveness in the specific machine and knowledge environment where they are to function. That conspectus, however, does not seem to be immediately forthcoming from modern departments of engineering, who seem to me to be concerned with vaster problems of utter generality. Therefore, those applied system designers who interest themselves in applications fields will apparently be forced to construct such limited theories for themselves.

If we model an EEG analysis study at a level which includes the investigator as data reducer, we see that even the linear methods mentioned above lead to threshold decisions, for example, "to mention or not to mention?" or "to interpret or not?" concerning particular features of the data which have been indicated by these linear methods. The nonlinear methods mentioned above are usually summarized by conventional statistics, which can in many cases be brought into a linear system format. Indeed, it is the appropriately hybridized methods which often give the most interesting scientific results; I would include as examples of this (analog) filtering followed by discriminant and other multivariate analyses (Fairchild et al., 1969), or the combination of spectra viewed as a linear system method, followed by threshold programs for classification (Viglione, or Larsen, *this volume;* Walter et al., 1967; Berkhout et al., 1969).

It seems that a useful tool would be a synthesis theory which included linear subsystems and memoryless nonlinear subsystems as its only available building blocks. This repertoire seems to cover many of our present systems: adders, amplifiers, low-, high- or band-pass filters, matched filters, integrator or differentiator circuits represent the usual linear set, whereas rectifiers, triggers, logic gates, squarers or multipliers are the usual memoryless nonlinear ones. There seems to exist an analysis and synthesis theory for black boxes assumed to be composed of such boxes: it was developed and applied by Spekreijse ("Analysis of EEG Responses in Man Evoked by Sine Wave Modulated Light," The Hague, Dr. W. Junk, 1966) to synthesize impressive models of visual evoked responses (for the method, see also *Kybernetick,* 7:22, 1970). Spekreijse's method may not be applicable to all problems in this class, since it appears to require either control of the input or else that the natural input be of a certain kind; but it is such a powerful and straightforward method that it is worth our study for those cases where it does apply. Perhaps Spekreijse himself or other system theorists would be able to extend those methods to various similar cases.

With such a theory available, we should no longer be limited to devices which can be imagined wholly at one blow, but could begin to synthesize more complex ones while still retaining some intuitive touch with the design process (unlike the loss of contact which I, at least, feel in trying to use some of the more advanced and generalized methods). For example, the cleverly applied matched filtering which is reported in this volume by Zetterberg was followed by a gate and threshold device to indicate probable presence of a sought transient: it applied to two channels the same sort of linear processing which has been applied to a single one by others. However, if the two channels have any coherence in the absence of the transient, then it seems likely that independent processing of the two is not the optimum detector. Here seems to be a clear example of linear systems (the matched filters) followed by memoryless nonlinear ones (the gate and threshold units), whose design might be noticeably improved by application of Spekreijse's theory, or an extension of it.

I must admit that both autocorrelators and phase-locked loops (see Nirenberg et al. for an EEG application) escape from this theory: clever devices are always ahead of general theory.

Another example of this mixture is complex demodulation in its usual form, which has multiplication by two preselected functions, followed by low-pass filtering, followed by memoryless r.m.s. operator in parallel with a memoryless inverse-tangent operator. Or another device which I suggested off the top of my head at the symposium for matched filtering is to dissect the sought transient into parts, seeking for them separately, and then announce occurrence of the transient, if several thresholds were surpassed in the proper time relation. It may be objected that this cannot do better than ordinary matched filtering, which is known to be optimum, at least for stationary Gaussian noise. But if the noise is far from stationary, or far from Gaussian in certain bands, or both, then we do not know how robust this proof may be. Even when the noise (read *background activity*) is nonstationary, it seems likely in EEG that its variations may be well represented by a slowly varying spectrum. Let me propose a descriptive model for plausible EEG nonstationariness which leads to a three-phase system design: let us make (Fig. 1) a factor analysis of the spectra of a subject's EEGs from one channel (Larsen has done this, among others); the factors can be principal components, or they can be some recondite rotation, orthogonal or not. Now construct filters (Fig. 2) whose attenuation curves match the weights assigned to various frequencies in each factor (that is, there will be as many

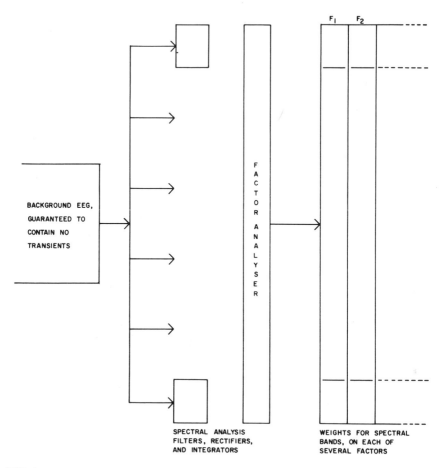

FIG. 1

filters as there were factors extracted). Pass the desired transient through those same filters, and note the output time histories. These components of the transient can then be used as a set of templates which are used in matched filtering (Fig. 3), while their integrated outputs are used for factor estimation. The probability that a component of the transient has been observed can be estimated from these two outputs from the same filter; hence an "and" gate combining the decisions about whether each component has occurred might be used to decide whether the whole transient has occurred.

But this system also falls into the category I have been describing, consisting of linear subsystems and memoryless nonlinear ones, so perhaps it, too, could be optimized by the design theory I have been discussing, although not producing.

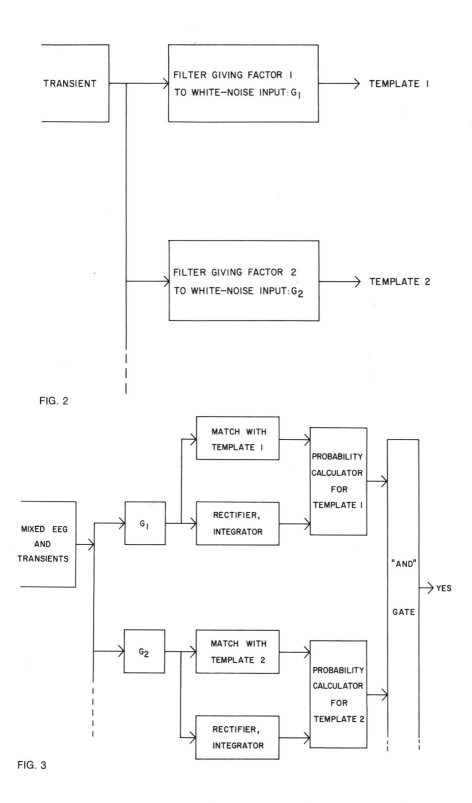

FIG. 2

FIG. 3

Automation of Clinical Electroencephalography.
Edited by P. Kellaway and I. Petersén.
Raven Press, New York © 1973.

A System for Transmitting Multichannel EEG Over the Public Telephone Network

K. E. Morander, R. Magnusson and I. Petersén

Department of Applied Electronics, Chalmers University of Technology, and Department of Clinical Neurophysiology, Sahlgren Hospital, Göteborg, Sweden

I. INTRODUCTION

A. Organization of Clinical EEG Service in Göteborg

In Göteborg, Sweden, the present organization of the visual interpretation of clinical EEG is based on a central laboratory at the university hospital (the Sahlgren Hospital) serving a number of peripheral laboratories. The physicians at the central laboratory interpret recordings not only from their own laboratory but from the peripheral laboratories as well, since these are not manned by doctors specializing in EEG. The recordings are sent from the peripheral laboratories by regular mail or by special messengers. At present, a total of about 12,000 recordings are interpreted each year.

It is obvious that transportation of the EEG recordings entails considerable cost as well as considerable loss of time. A further drawback of the system is that the registrations are available as ink recordings only. Although methods now exist for regaining the electrical signal by means of curve readers (Lindholm and Petersén, 1970, 1972), such methods necessarily entail some loss of signal quality. A possible alternative is to record the EEG signals on magnetic tape at each laboratory, but such a procedure would be quite expensive.

B. Advantages of EEG Telemetry

Telemetry of EEG signals from the peripheral laboratories to the central laboratory would not only obviate the need for record transportation, yielding gains in reduced cost and reduced transmission time, but would probably also render possible reduction of peripheral laboratory staff. It is reasonable to expect that a single EEG technician equipped with a single EEG machine could monitor and comment upon the EEGs of several patients being investigated simultaneously. The EEG machine would be used for checking the transmitted EEGs only and not for recording them. Even disregarding a future automated interpretation of the recordings, it should be possible to gain in objectivity and diagnostic reliability if the idea of a central laboratory can be realized. At the proposed EEG Center, a large number of EEG physicians sharing a pool of great experience will be on duty, and consultation with colleagues on any doubtful cases will be expedient. It is likely, however, that the most important benefit of introducing telemetry is the possibility provided for peripheral EEG stations lacking EEG experts to obtain rapid diagnostic information.

C. EEG Telemetry in Göteborg

The planning and development of a central, automated EEG laboratory in Göteborg has now been in progress for nearly a decade. As the project developed, it became evident that, since adequate systems were not commercially available, the telemetry problem would have to be solved by our own group – the Neuronics Group, consisting of the Department of Applied Electronics at Chalmers University of Technology, the Department of Clinical Neurophysiology at Sahlgren Hospital, and Kaisers Laboratorium A/S. In 1968 we started the development of a system for transmission over the public telephone network of EEG recordings containing at least eight channels. The project has now reached a stage at which several test transmissions over considerable distances have been successfully performed. At present, the results of a series of transmissions from Lillhagen Hospital to Sahlgren Hospital – a distance of about 13 km – are being evaluated. The transmitting laboratory at Lillhagen Hospital is shown in Fig. 1.

To our knowledge, no long-distance transmissions of complete EEG recordings (containing at least eight channels) over the public telephone network have been reported. At Karolinska Hospital in Stockholm, eight-channel EEG is transmitted within the hospital area (Ottoson and Persson, 1970). The system makes use of 10 pairs of wires running together, into which the amplified EEG signals are entered; in other words, no modulation

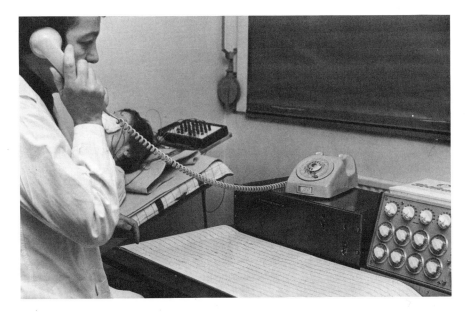

FIG. 1. Telemetry transmitter at Lillhagen Hospital.

procedure is employed. In the United States, Bennet and Gardner (1970) have reported transmissions of six-channel EEG. The modulating and demodulating equipment employed by these authors necessitates the use of two parallel lines.

II. ENGINEERING ASPECTS OF EEG TELEMETRY

A. Number of Channels

At the present time, a slight trend to favor 16-channel recordings over eight-channel recordings can be noted. It should also be noted, however, that the main advantage of the 16-channel system is some saving of time in recording the EEG. There are several reasons opposing the use of 16-channel recordings, such as bulkiness, less clear presentation, more expensive tape recordings and, as far as telemetry is concerned, considerable engineering problems due to limited telephone-line bandwidth. To some extent, the bandwidth problems can be overcome by using direct-coupled, rented lines. This method becomes uneconomical, however, when longer distances are involved.

In view of the present uncertainty about the future preference with regard to the number of channels recorded, it has been our goal to develop a system which (1) is capable of transmitting eight channels over the public telephone network, and (2) can be easily expanded to accommodate 16 channels in case rented lines are used.

B. Transmission System

Owing to pen inertia, EEG recorded by galvanometer pens has an upper cut-off frequency of approximately 30 to 40 Hz. Transmission bandwidths of some 40 Hz per channel should thus be sufficient to ensure adequate visual interpretation of the curves. Presently available computerized methods of analysis, such as correlation and power spectrum analyses, are applied to signals having bandwidths of approximately 30 Hz. Of the immediately interesting methods of automatic analysis, only those involving automatic pattern recognition may require bandwidths in excess of 30 Hz, primarily because pattern recognition schemes — still quite limited in number — require high-quality transient response in order to retain spike information. With these various requirements in mind, we decided to aim at a transmission bandwidth of approximately 50 Hz per channel.

The modulator-demodulator equipment supplied by the Swedish Telecommunications Administration yields transmission speeds of at most 1,200 bauds over the public telephone network, and at most 4,800 bauds over rented lines. Transmission of a 50-Hz wide signal requires a lowest sampling frequency of, in theory, $2 \times 50 = 100$ Hz. A practical sampling frequency might be 150 Hz. For reproduction of the EEG signal we may require, say, 100 levels of quantization, corresponding to about seven bits in a digital code. The data transmission channel must thus be capable of handling $7 \times 150 = 1,050$ bauds. In order to transmit a complete EEG recording in real time, we thus need eight parallel modems, each with a transmission speed of 1,200 bauds. Although the telephone lines themselves may permit vastly higher transmission speeds, at least over the local network, the usable range is limited by interference susceptibility as well as by government regulations. We must resort to a frequency-division multiplex system.

The frequency range available on the telephone lines is 600 to 2,100 Hz. In an eight-channel system, approximately 190 Hz can thus be allotted to each channel. In the case of amplitude modulation retaining both sidebands, the bandwidth of the signal is 100 Hz. The frequency interval between the upper sideband of a channel and the lower sideband of the next higher-frequency channel thus is 90 Hz, corresponding to a relative channel separation of some 5% at the highest channel. In other words, channel separation will require quite steep cut-off filters. Realization of these filters does not present too much of a design problem if modern active-filter technique is used. In fact, as far as selection-filter realization is concerned, the channels could be placed considerably closer. The main problem encountered when increasing filter selectivity is that the transient response of the filter deteriorates to a corresponding degree. Rapid signal changes become accompanied by large and slowly decaying overshoots.

A second problem encountered in telemetry over the telephone network is caused by impulse disturbances created by time markers and dial operations. These disturbances frequently have amplitudes of 10 times the maximum permissible signal amplitude. Since they essentially are impulses, they have a very wide power spectrum. The influence of these disturbances can be reduced by means of a frequency-modulation frequency-division multiplex system, in which each EEG signal modulates the frequency of its own carrier oscillator. As shown in Fig. 2, the oscillator output signals are summed and entered into the line. A typical shape of the resulting composite signal in the case of eight equidistant carrier waves is shown in Fig. 3. Owing to the small bandwidth available per channel, frequency modulation will be of the narrow-band type. In other words, at the highest modulation frequencies—approximately 50 Hz—only the two sidebands closest to the carrier will be transmitted.

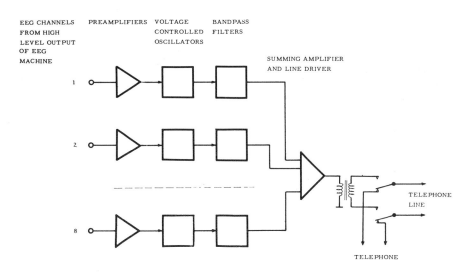

FIG. 2. Eight-channel EEG transmitter.

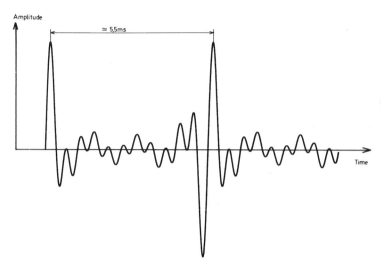

FIG. 3. Typical frequency-division multiplex signal consisting of eight carrier waves of equal distances.

III. AN EIGHT-CHANNEL TELEMETRY SYSTEM

In this section we give a brief description of our present eight-channel, frequency-modulation, frequency-division multiplex telemetry system. In order to accommodate two extra channels for future transmission of heart frequency and eye movements (or any two low-frequency signals), a carrier frequency spacing of 180 Hz has been chosen. The frequency disposition is shown in Fig. 4.

One of our goals has been to develop a system of sufficiently low complexity to ensure acceptable cost when the system is introduced on a larger

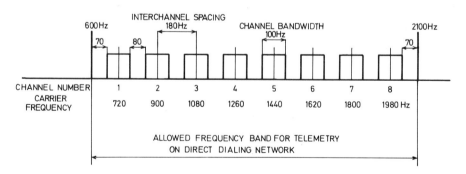

FIG. 4. Frequency spacing of eight-channel telemetry system.

scale. Thus, the carrier-frequency oscillators consist of simple square-wave generators. The output of each oscillator is filtered in an active bandpass filter having a Butterworth selectivity curve of the type shown in Fig. 5. These filters suppress square-wave harmonics as well as nondesirable modulation sidebands. The filter output signals are essentially pure sinusoids. As illustrated in Fig. 2, the eight carriers are then added in a summing amplifier, which also serves to drive the line transformer.

A block diagram of the receiving equipment is shown in Fig. 6. The composite signal is first amplified, and then entered into active bandpass filters separating the channels. The filters are of third-order Chebyshev type with a passband ripple of ± 0.25 dB. Some representative selectivity curves are shown in Fig. 7. The separated carriers are amplitude limited, and the modulating signal is regained in phase-lock detectors. This type of detector, shown in Fig. 8, has proved to have an excellent ability to suppress impulse disturbances. In brief, it operates as follows. The phase θ_i of the input signal is compared to the phase θ_o of a locally generated signal. If the two signal frequencies coincide, the phase detector output contains a DC component which is a measure of the phase difference $\theta_i - \theta_o$. This DC component, the output of the lowpass "loop filter," is used to control the frequency of the locally generated signal, so that its phase θ_o continually follows the input signal phase θ_i. Now, if the transmitter oscillator and the receiver oscillator are equal, the two voltages controlling them must also be equal. The loop-filter output signal thus is the demodulated EEG signal. Carrier frequency remnants are suppressed in a third-order, lowpass post-detection filter.

The system fulfills the Swedish requirements on equipment to be con-

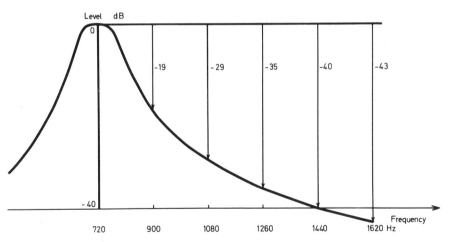

FIG. 5. Bandpass characteristics of the transmitter filter.

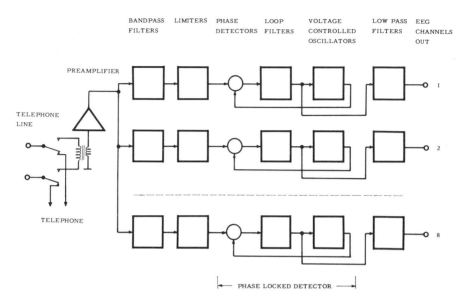

FIG. 6. Eight-channel EEG receiver.

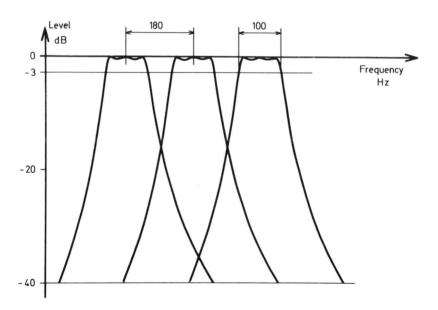

FIG. 7. Bandpass characteristics of the receiver filters.

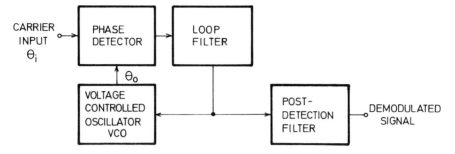

FIG. 8. Phase-lock FM discriminator.

nected to the public telephone network. These requirements essentially state that the system shall be matched to a line impedance of 600 ohms, that the transmitted power must not exceed 0.1 mW into 600 ohms in the frequency range 600 to 2,100 Hz, and that the power of any signal components in the range above 2,100 Hz shall be less than −34 dBm.

Each EEG channel has an overall bandwidth of 45 Hz, and an overshoot in the overall step-function response of 5%.

IV. PRACTICAL EXPERIENCE WITH THE EIGHT-CHANNEL SYSTEM

The system described above was first tested, with satisfactory results, on a 2-km long, rented standard line between Chalmers University of Technology and Sahlgren Hospital. With the kind assistance of the Swedish Telecommunications Administration, we have also tested the system over a standard-line connection from Göteborg to Stockholm and back, a distance of 1,000 km. Here, too, the results were good. Figure 9 shows the signal received when a sinusoid of frequency 40 Hz was transmitted.

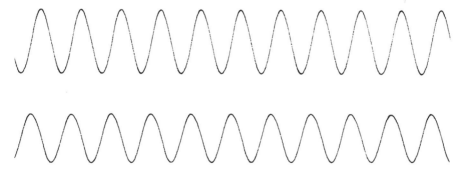

FIG. 9. 1000 km transmission of 40-Hz signal. *Upper trace:* transmitted 40-Hz sinusoid. *Lower trace:* received signal.

At present, the system is being clinically tested in transmissions from Lill-hagen Hospital to Sahlgren Hospital. As mentioned above, the distance is 13 km. The experience so far has been good. Figure 10 shows a typical example of recordings from a patient. The lower eight traces are signals recorded in the central laboratory at Sahlgren Hospital. Owing to the 45-Hz transmission bandwidth, occasionally appearing high-frequency myoelectric

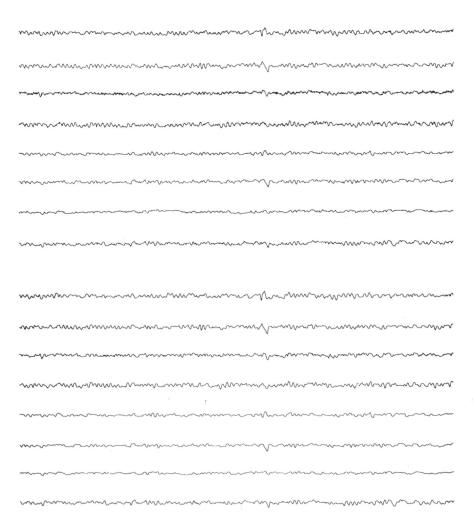

FIG. 10. Simultaneous recordings of eight-channel EEG at Lillhagen Hospital and at Sahlgren Hospital. *Upper eight curves:* transmitted EEG. *Lower eight curves:* received EEG.

signals are suppressed. Apart from this, the curves contain no visually discernible differences.

V. ECONOMICAL ASPECTS

If the cost of one transmitter plus one receiver is assumed to be $6,000 each, the annual capital cost, for an equipment life of 10 years, will be about $1,200. For connections over the local network, this will be essentially the only expense item, since EEG machines, laboratory space, etc., must be available whether telemetry is used or not. An alternative to single-line telemetry is to use 10 rented parallel pairs of wires, together with a simple line matching unit. The estimated costs per year and kilometer for these two alternative systems are shown in Fig. 11. As evident from the diagram,

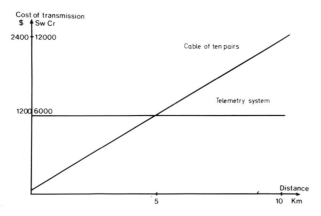

FIG. 11. Annual cost vs. distance for EEG transmission over the local network: (a) multiplex system, (b) system using ten DC-coupled wire pairs in parallel.

rented lines are more economical for distances less than 5 km. In some regions, limited availability of wire pairs for rent may be a decisive factor.

If the direct dialing system is to be used over longer distances, connection-time costs will rapidly become dominating. This is illustrated by the staircase curve in Fig. 12. An economically better solution is to rent a standard line. Assuming the system is used 8 hr a day for 220 days a year, one can estimate the annual number of transmitted EEGs to be about 1,000. For very large distances, of the order of 450 km, the transmission cost per EEG will then be about $13. These estimations are based on Swedish tariffs. Bennet and Gardner (1970) have published a corresponding estimation based on their

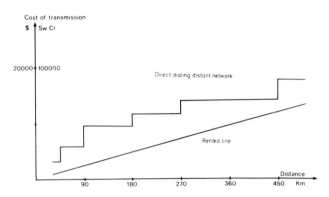

FIG. 12. Annual cost vs. distance for EEG transmission over the long-distance network: (a) direct-dialing system, (b) system using a rented line.

system, six-channel EEG using two lines over a distance of 400 km, and on American tariffs, with the result of $36 per EEG.

VI. FUTURE DEVELOPMENTS

The present eight-channel system is now being expanded to accommodate another two channels for transmitting slowly varying signals, such as eye movements and respiration or heart frequency. We have also found that the system should permit backward signaling from the receiving central laboratory to the transmitting peripheral laboratory. In order to give information on electrode configurations as well as comments on the EEG tracings, the technician at the peripheral laboratory at present has to interrupt the transmission and establish voice contact with the receiving technician. This is a further respect in which the system can be improved. It is not very difficult, for instance, to have the peripheral laboratory recorder control the paper feed of the receiving recorder, and to code standard information digitally for transmission simultaneously with the EEG.

Our present system is a laboratory prototype. We have hopes that an industrial version will become available in the near future, rendering more extensive clinical tests possible.

DISCUSSION

In response to several discussants who questioned the extent to which cross-talk between channels had been encountered, Magnusson said that this had not proved to be a problem. Walter suggested that the bandwidth of 45 Hz might allow transmission of a record which would be suitable for visual analysis, but that more refined types of analysis might not be possible. Zetterberg agreed with this comment, pointing out that some of the analysis techniques that he had described would probably require a larger bandwidth. Magnusson replied that the system that he had described was a prototype, and these and other aspects would have to be thoroughly checked out.

Discussion then turned to the possibility of using other transmission techniques. Coaxial cables would be satisfactory within a medical center. Microwave transmission would provide adequate bandwidth but would be costly in most applications, and it would probably prove difficult to have a channel allocated for EEG transmission only. Saltzberg mentioned that digital data transmission systems are becoming more widely used, and if a digital network were installed primarily for some other reason but became relatively inexpensively available for EEG transmission, this would open up new possibilities.

In response to a question from Zetterberg, Magnusson said that they had found no difference in the noise between the rented line and the direct-dialing method.

REFERENCES

Bennet, D. R. and Gardner, R. M. (1970): A model for the telephone transmission of six-channel electroencephalograms. *Electroencephalography and Clinical Neurophysiology,* 29:404–408.

Lindholm, L.-E. and Petersén, I. (1970): An ink-trace follower for the conversion of graphical records to analog electrical signals. *Proceedings of the First Nordic Meeting on Medical and Biological Engineering.*

Lindholm, L.-E. and Petersén, I.: A simple and inexpensive curve reader for high speed reconversion of ink recordings to electrical signals. Institute of Electrical and Electronics Engineers Transactions on Bio-Medical Engineering (*in press*).

Ottoson, S. and Persson, A. (1970): Transmission of EEG within a hospital area. (*In Swedish.*) *Elektronik,* 12:61–62.